Heart Sounds Made Easy

For Elsevier
Commissioning Editor: Laurence Hunter
Development Editor: Helen Leng
Project Manager: Christine Johnston
Design Direction: Erik Bigland
Illustrator: Robert Britton
Illustration Manager: Gillian Richards

Heart Sounds Made Easy

Second edition

Elspeth M Brown MB ChB FRCPCH
Consultant Paediatric Cardiologist
Leeds General Infirmary, Leeds, UK

Terence S Leung PhD MSc BEng
Senior Research Fellow
Department of Medical Physics and Bioengineering
University College London, UK

William B Collis PhD BEng
Associate Fellow
Institute of Sound and Vibration Research
University of Southampton, UK

Anthony P Salmon FRCP FRCPCH
Consultant Congenital Cardiologist
Wessex Cardiothoracic Centre
Southampton General Hospital
Southampton, UK

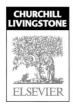

Edinburgh London New York Oxford Philadelphia St Louis Sydney Toronto 2008

CHURCHILL LIVINGSTONE
ELSEVIER

An imprint of Elsevier Limited

© 2002, 2008, Elsevier Limited. All rights reserved.

First edition 2002
Second edition 2008
  Reprinted 2009, 2010 (twice), 2012, 2013 (twice), 2014

ISBN: 9780443069079

British Library Cataloguing in Publication Data
A catalogue record for this book is available from the British Library

Library of Congress Cataloging in Publication Data
A catalog record for this book is available from the Library of Congress

Note

Neither the publisher nor the authors assume any responsibility for any loss or injury and/or damage to persons or property arising out of or related to any use of the material contained in this book. It is the responsibility of the treating practitioner, relying on independent expertise and knowledge of the patient, to determine the best treatment and method of application for the patient.

The Publisher

your source for books,
journals and multimedia
in the health sciences

www.elsevierhealth.com

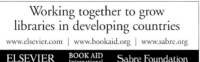

Working together to grow
libraries in developing countries

www.elsevier.com | www.bookaid.org | www.sabre.org

The
publisher's
policy is to use
**paper manufactured
from sustainable forests**

Reprinted with permission by Elsevier Australia for
Servier Laboratories (Australia) Pty Ltd, 2009.
Printed in China.

Preface

Cardiac auscultation is one of the most difficult skills to acquire and competence in this area is extremely variable. Teaching is traditionally carried out at the bedside, with an expert describing the physical signs and the trainee nodding knowingly. The main skill acquired is the ability to appear knowledgeable while remaining mystified. This method of teaching does not allow the trainer or trainee to verify that they are appreciating the specific auscultatory features in the different parts of the cardiac cycle. We want to give you the opportunity to learn auscultation skills as if you have a consultant cardiologist present to teach you at your convenience. This is a short and accessible book that takes you through the questions that we ask ourselves when listening to heart sounds. It can be used alone or in conjunction with the CD of heart sounds recorded from actual patients.

The *Heart Sounds Made Easy* CD is an interactive tool based on the latest digital audio technology. It allows users to listen to a recording and either eliminate or enhance the different components until they are confident that they have correctly identified the sounds in all phases of the cardiac cycle. This is particularly important for the recognition of diastolic sounds which are the most difficult to appreciate. There is no better way to confirm the presence of such a murmur than to have the facility to reduce or increase its intensity. This software is now used routinely for teaching auscultation to students and junior doctors on the Wessex Cardiothoracic Unit in Southampton, where it has proved successful and popular.

In the five years since the first edition of the book was published, computer software has changed considerably and so we felt we needed to update our CD. This has allowed us to add new features, such as the ability to slow the heart sounds down without altering their pitch. We have also changed the layout of the CD to make it easier to access. We have added questions and answers in the book and on the CD to allow readers to monitor their knowledge and progress. The visual representation of the cardiac cycle will also allow readers to understand the origin of the heart sounds. We hope that you find the book and CD are a useful educational aid.

Southampton   E.M.B.
2008   T.L.
                                                                                                 W.C.
                                                                                               A.P.S.

Acknowledgements

First and foremost we wish to thank all the patients and their families for allowing us to record their heart sounds. We must also thank the staff and trustees of Wessex Heartbeat for all their support in developing the heart sound manipulator and providing the funds to help develop this technology and CD. We would like to express our particular gratitude to Alan Prince who, as chairman of Wessex Heartbeat Trustees, maintained the momentum necessary for the completion of the first edition of the book and CD. Our thanks to Paul White, Antonello de Stefano and Alfredo Giani at the Institute of Sound and Vibration Research at Southampton University for their help in developing the CD software for the first edition.

Contents

How to use the book and CD

The *Heart Sounds Made Easy* book and CD can be used together or separately. Each chapter of the book corresponds to a region of the chest and the corresponding sounds. For each heart sound you should read the information in the relevant chapter to familiarize yourself with the anatomy, history, examination and characteristics of a particular heart sound. You should then listen to the relevant tutorial on the CD.

The CD is best listened to through high-quality headphones or good-quality speakers. Listening through headphones gives an experience closer to that of listening through a stethoscope than does using speakers. The PC version requires a 1.4 Ghz processor or better. On inserting the CD into your PC it should start automatically. If not, choose My Computer, and double click the *start* icon on the CD drive. For the Macintosh, insert the CD into the CD drive and double click on the *macstart* icon.

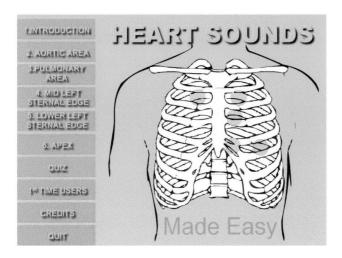

The initial main menu screen allows you to choose the *1ˢᵗ TIME USERS* button, which leads to an introduction to the aims of the CD. The *CREDITS* button gives information on the organizations involved in producing the CD and book.

This screen also shows the contents, containing chapter headings that correspond with those in the book. Choose the area you are interested in and click on the button. You will then see a screen that shows a list of the heart sounds best heard in that area (see illustration overleaf). This corresponds to the sounds discussed in that chapter of the book. Choose the heart sound you are interested in and the interactive software will be launched.

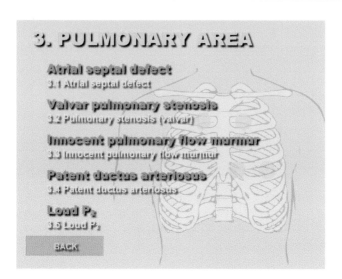

On starting the interactive software, the selected heart sound will be played automatically. There are two main panels (see opposite). The upper one (the manipulator) allows the user to adjust the volume of individual components of the selected heart sound, such as the first heart sound (S_1), the second heart sound (S_2), the systolic and diastolic components. Note that these components are colour coded on the phonocardiogram, with the colour corresponding to the volume sliders below. Under the volume sliders you will also notice that two circular cursors are flashing in synchronization with the heart sound. The red cursor is on during systole while the blue cursor is on during diastole. These cursors provide visual timings of systole and diastole and are referred to as the systolic and diastolic cursors (SDC) in the book and in the tutorial of the interactive software.

An animation of the heart is also displayed in synchronization with the heart sound. The red and blue arrows correspond to the flow of blood in the left and right chambers of the heart. Blue arrows are used to indicate the location where audible murmurs are caused. For heart sounds associated with a problematic heart valve, e.g. the pulmonary valve in pulmonary stenosis, the heart valve is highlighted in red.

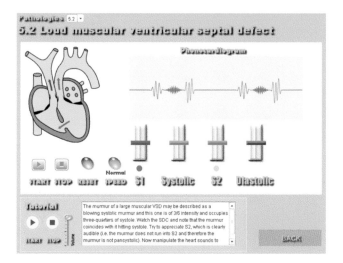

Below the animation are two buttons for starting and stopping the heart sound and animation. The *RESET* button can be used to re-adjust the volumes of the four components of the heart sound to their original levels. The *SPEED* button allows the heart sound to toggle between the normal and slow speeds. The slowed version of the heart sound enables the users to appreciate the subtle characteristics of the heart sound and has been digitally processed so that the sound is slowed down while keeping the same pitch.

The lower panel is for the tutorial. On clicking the *START* button, the instructor's voice can be heard and the text version of the instruction will also be displayed. During a tutorial, each component of the heart sound will be automatically adjusted according to the context of the tutorial. Users who prefer to focus on the heart sound rather than the instructor's voice can minimize the voice volume using the volume slider.

At the top of the screen, there is a pull-down menu allowing the users to switch to a different heart sound. There is also a *BACK* button on the lower right corner of the screen to go back to the main menu.

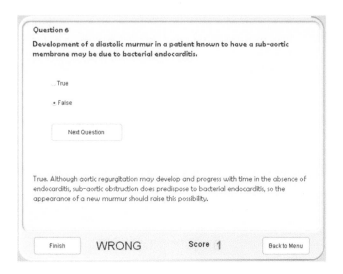

Question 6

Development of a diastolic murmur in a patient known to have a sub-aortic membrane may be due to bacterial endocarditis.

  True

• False

Next Question

True. Although aortic regurgitation may develop and progress with time in the absence of endocarditis, sub-aortic obstruction does predispose to bacterial endocarditis, so the appearance of a new murmur should raise this possibility.

Finish   WRONG   Score 1   Back to Menu

An interactive quiz is available for users to test their knowledge on heart sound auscultation and can be started from the main menu. There are a total of 170 questions which are extracted from the quiz sections of the book. The quiz can be terminated at any time by clicking the *Finish* button and a score will be displayed.

Introduction

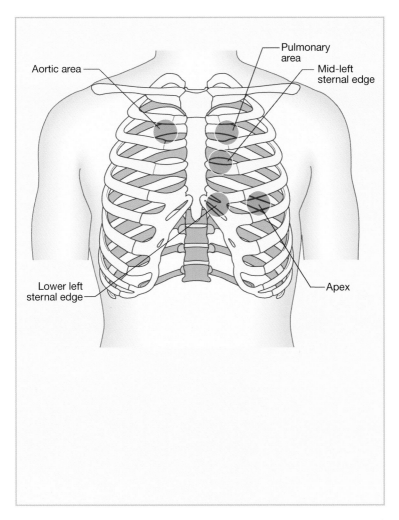

Aortic area

Pulmonary area

Mid-left sternal edge

Lower left sternal edge

Apex

Listening to the heart and recognizing normal and abnormal sounds is a skill necessary to many health professionals. The heart, perhaps more than any other organ, may reveal abnormalities on examination in an otherwise asymptomatic individual. The ability to differentiate the abnormal from the normal, and to make an assessment of the need for, and urgency of, investigation is therefore vital to all health professionals involved in frontline patient care. This said however, it is still as important as ever to take a thorough clinical history and perform a full general examination to put these findings in context. In this chapter we will cover the features of the history and examination that are particularly pertinent to diseases of the heart. Specific investigation will be briefly discussed but for a more thorough discussion of the investigation and treatment of cardiac disease the reader is referred to one of the much larger and comprehensive textbooks on cardiology.

History

Although there are a large number of cardiovascular diseases, there are only a handful of possible symptoms.

Pain

Exertional chest pain is most frequently associated with coronary artery disease, but hypertrophic cardiomyopathy and severe outflow tract obstruction may result in cardiac pain. The pain is typically situated in the upper chest and described as tight or crushing. It may be experienced as a feeling of breathlessness. The pain may radiate down the left arm or into the jaw. In angina the pain typically occurs during exercise, and is relieved by rest or nitrates. In a myocardial infarction, the pain is more severe and prolonged and is not relieved by these measures. There may be accompanying nausea, vomiting or sweating. Such pain must be differentiated from pain arising from the upper GI tract, and the relation to exercise and relieving factors aid in this. Other pain associated with cardiac disease is the sharp central pain of pericarditis. This is exacerbated with deep breathing and on leaning forward. Dissection of the thoracic aorta leads to a severe pain, often felt between the shoulder blades at the back.

Breathlessness

Breathlessness is another important symptom of cardiac disease, and must be differentiated from breathlessness due to pulmonary disease, although the two may coexist. Breathlessness is initially confined to exertion but in severe disease is present at rest. This however is also the case in pulmonary disease. A history of orthopnoea or paroxysmal nocturnal dyspnoea is highly suggestive of cardiac as opposed to respiratory disease, although it may require further investigation to determine confidently the source of the symptom.

Palpitations

Palpitations are a frequent symptom in the population and usually represent only an awareness of normal sinus tachycardia, or of premature beats. However, palpitations related to arrhythmias may be the presenting feature of many different cardiac conditions, including structural heart disease, ischaemic heart disease and cardiomyopathy, as well as a primary arrhythmia.

Syncope in the population is most commonly vasovagal in origin but this is a diagnosis of exclusion, as syncope may reflect life-threatening cardiac disease, including severe outflow tract obstruction, cardiomyopathy or arrhythmia.

Swelling of the ankles due to dependent oedema is frequently not associated with cardiac disease but is a feature of congestive cardiac failure.

Further history

With better understanding of the genetic causes of heart disease, both ischaemic and non-ischaemic, a detailed family history, focussing on known heart disease, congenital and acquired, and sudden death in a family member is mandatory. Increasingly, patients are being investigated because of their family history, either of a condition with a known genetic cause, or because of sudden death at a young age where no cause was found on post-mortem examination, raising the possibility of a primary cardiac dysrhythmia. Obviously patients in the first category are easier to investigate than those in the latter, although even when a genetic defect is known it may be impossible to be completely reassuring.

The patient's previous general health and lifestyle are also important. Patients with congenital heart disease, such as an atrial septal defect, may take for granted that they have always had less stamina than their peers. A previous history of murmur or investigation for possible heart disease can be very illuminating.

The patient's smoking history and previous drug ingestion, both prescribed and recreational, may have a bearing on their current cardiac health.

A previous history of rheumatic fever should be specifically sought, as should a history of diabetes. The patient should also be asked about the amount of exercise that they routinely take now, and have taken in the past, as this may well uncover a slow deterioration in symptoms. Enquiries should be made as to whether the patient has a history of systemic hypertension, and whether they know their lipid profile.

Examination

As with all physical examination, it is important to have the patient fully undressed. However, the patient's dignity must be respected at all times and leaving them exposed unnecessarily should be avoided. When examining children it is some-times the case that trying to get them undressed may upset them so much that it is impossible to listen to them and compromise is therefore necessary. The same is true with regard to getting a child into the perfect position for an exami-nation, and a more flexible approach may be necessary, sometimes with the examination repeated at a later date.

General physical examination

General examination will include assessment of the height and weight of the patient, together with calculation of the body mass index (BMI). Obesity is an important risk factor for ischaemic heart disease, and is an added stress on any patient with cardiovascular disease, be it congenital or acquired. Extremes of stature, either short or tall, may suggest a possible syndrome associated with cardiac disease, and careful examination looking for possible features is necessary, particularly in the skeletal and gastrointestinal systems. A strong suspicion of a possible syndrome may require further investigation to demonstrate diagnostic features. Certain forms of congenital heart disease (those with a significant left to right shunt, and those associated with severe cyanosis) may lead to impaired growth in childhood. This has been reduced by the trend to earlier surgical cor-rection of amenable lesions in developed countries; however, older patients, and those from the developing world, may still show growth restriction.

The skin should be examined for xanthelasmas, which are an important sign of raised serum cholesterol. The presence of peripheral and central cyanosis should be sought, and the oxygen saturation measured by pulse oximetry where this is available. A clinical assessment of anaemia should be made, as well as noting if the patient may be polycythaemic, as occurs with long-standing cyanosis. Finger clubbing, and the presence and extent of oedema should be noted. The presence of pleural effusion or ascites should be sought, particularly if there is peripheral oedema.

Cardiovascular examination

Abnormalities of the features which relate to specific pathologies will be discussed in the following chapters with the murmurs which relate to that condition. Some general points will be considered here.

Arterial pulsation/blood pressure

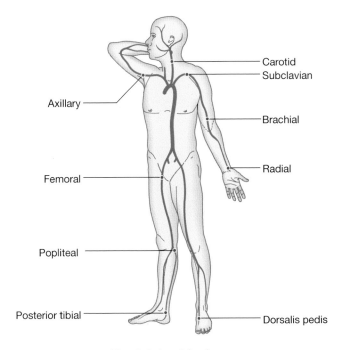

Fig. 1.1 *Arterial pulses*

The radial pulse is initially assessed for rate and rhythm with the patient sitting or reclining comfortably. If the rate is irregular, an assessment of the heart rate by listening at the apex should be compared to the pulse rate at the wrist and the *pulse deficit* noted. The character and volume are classically assessed at the carotid pulse, but, particularly in children, this may be distressing and the brachial pulse may be used. All the pulses should be palpated and the volume compared with the other side (not simultaneously in the case of the carotid pulse). The radial and femoral pulses should also be compared to detect the presence of radiofemoral delay or a weakness in the femoral pulse in coarctation. The difference between the systolic and diastolic blood pressure measured with a sphygmomanometer gives an important objective measure of pulse pressure. Appropriate choice of blood pressure cuff is vital for obtaining an accurate reading, and the accurate measurement of blood pressure is covered in textbooks of clinical examination.

Venous pulsation

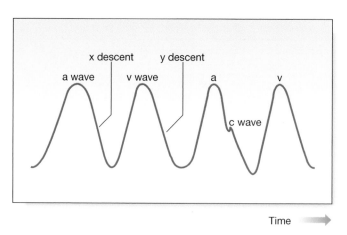

Fig. 1.2 *The normal venous pulse*

The central venous pulse is assessed with the patient lying comfortably at 45° and the height is described as centimetres above the clavicle. In normal patients the jugular venous pulse is not visible. It may be very difficult to assess, particularly in obese patients, or in infants who have short necks and increased subcutaneous fat. A raised jugular venous pressure is an important sign of cardiac failure, or obstruction to the superior vena cava, in which case pulsation is lost. The venous pulse has an A wave due to atrial contraction and a V wave due to the rise in atrial pressure during ventricular systole. A smaller C wave is not usually visible in the neck but represents onset of ventricular systole. There is an X and Y descent. All parts of the venous pulsation are only visible if the patient is in sinus rhythm.

Inspection of the chest

The chest should be inspected for signs of deformity, visible pulsation, enlarged veins and scars from previous surgery. Deformity such as kyphoscoliosis will affect the cardiac impulse and may lead to murmurs despite a structurally normal heart. In thin individuals the apex beat may be visible.

Palpation of the chest

The chest is palpated to determine the position of the cardiac apex, which is the lowest and outermost point where the cardiac pulsation is felt. The patient must be lying or sitting straight. In healthy individuals it will be in the mid-clavicular line, in the 5th intercostal space on the left. The position of the apex may be affected by the heart being displaced in the chest due to spine and rib deformities or lung disease, as well as cardiac disease. For example, a pleural effusion or pneumothorax will push the apex beat towards the contralateral side. If the apex is difficult to define, do not forget to palpate on the right side of the chest for dextrocardia. The quality of the apex beat should be assessed but this is affected by subcutaneous fat. The apex should also be felt to check for thrills. The chest should then be palpated using the flat of the hand on the left and right of the sternum to feel for a right ventricular heave (*left of sternum*) and thrills on either side. The suprasternal notch is palpated to check for an aortic thrill.

Percussion of the chest

The cardiac dullness may be percussed but in practice this is not routinely done. Percussion of the chest is more useful to confirm liver size, and if significant pleural effusions are present.

Auscultation

> **Remember**
> - Heart sounds
> - Added sounds
> - Murmurs

This is the main focus of this book and will be covered in detail in the following chapters. However here it is important to note that initially it is common to listen to the precordium and hope for inspiration to strike! A more fruitful approach is to listen systematically throughout the cardiac cycle. This will be referred to throughout the rest of the book but in essence it involves:

Heart sounds
First heart sound
Identify the first and second heart sounds and time using the carotid pulse if you are unsure. The first heart sound coincides with the carotid pulse. Listen to the first heart sound and decide if it appears loud, quiet or split. The first heart sound is not usually audibly split, despite the fact that it represents the closure of the mitral and tricuspid valves and these two events are not completely synchronous.

Second heart sound
Listen to the second sound and try to appreciate the normal variability of splitting with respiration. The second heart sound is caused by closure of the aortic and then pulmonary valves and the splitting can usually be appreciated, although not if the patient is tachycardic. If necessary ask the patient to breathe in deeply and hold their breath (if they are able to). If the second sound does not seem normal ask yourself is the second sound loud or soft, is it single, widely split and mobile, or widely split and fixed.

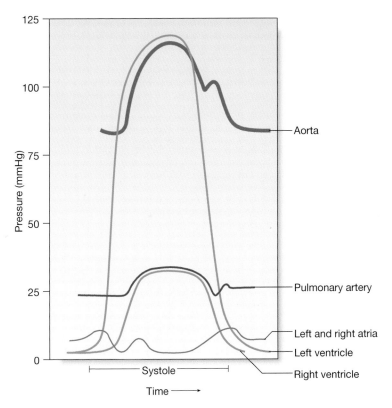

Fig. 1.3 *The cardiac cycle*

Next, listen for added sounds. These are ejection valve clicks after the first heart sound, an opening snap in late diastole, a third or a fourth heart sound. More than one extra sound may be present.

Added sounds
Third and fourth heart sounds
The third heart sound occurs in early diastole at the time of maximum ventricular filling. It may be heard in young fit adults and during pregnancy. The fourth heart sound occurs at the time of atrial contraction and is therefore only present

if the patient is in sinus rhythm. Both these sounds are best heard with the bell of the stethoscope and with the patient turned slightly onto the left side.

Clicks and snaps

The opening of a normal heart valve is silent. Ejection clicks arise from an abnormal aortic or pulmonary valve as it opens, and occur early in systole. They may be mistaken for splitting of the first heart sound. A prolapsing mitral valve may lead to a mid systolic click, which may be intermittent. An opening snap arises from an abnormal mitral or tricuspid valve and therefore is heard in diastole. Note that as the valve becomes more severely affected and the movement is decreased the click or snap will disappear.

Knock and rub

In constrictive pericarditis there may be a loud, low-frequency diastolic noise known as a knock. A pericardial rub is a high-frequency noise, loudest in systole, but often present in diastole as well. A rub may vary from hour to hour, and if a significant effusion develops the rub will disappear.

Finally, listen in systole and then in diastole for murmurs.

Murmurs

The timing of a murmur (systolic or diastolic) may be difficult, particularly if the patient is tachycardic. Systole may be timed by feeling the carotid pulse in the neck. Murmurs are systolic, diastolic, systolic and diastolic or continuous. The timing of murmurs is discussed in the relevant chapters.

Murmurs may be low pitched, such as mitral stenosis, or high pitched, such as small ventricular septal defects (VSDs). Murmurs vary in intensity but it is important to note that loud murmurs do not necessarily indicate severe disease. For example, small VSDs may give loud murmurs, whereas large ones may produce no murmur. Systolic murmurs are traditionally graded out of 6, with a 1/6 murmur being quiet and a 6/6 being very loud. Diastolic murmurs are graded out of four.

It is also important to determine whether the murmur changes during respiration. Typically, murmurs arising from the right heart are accentuated on inspiration.

It is important to follow this sequence at each position on the precordium and at the back. It is also important to recognize which abnormal signs tend to go together so that they may be specifically sought. So for example, a bicuspid aortic valve may be associated with a systolic ejection click which is best heard at the apex, a systolic aortic stenotic murmur which is best heard at the upper right sternal edge and a diastolic aortic regurgitation murmur which is best heard at the mid left sternal edge. The detection of any of these findings should lead to a careful listen for the presence of the others.

Table 1.1 Grading of systolic murmurs

Grade	Thrill	Murmur
1/6	Absent	Very quiet
2/6	Absent	Quiet
3/6	Absent	Easily audible
4/6	Present	Loud
5/6	Present	Audible with stethoscope half off chest
6/6	Present	Audible without stethoscope

Stethoscope

A high-quality stethoscope is an important investment and most can last a lifetime. The authors feel that an adult cardiological stethoscope is suitable for *all* ages (apart from premature neonates) and that these have better acoustic features than the smaller paediatric and neonatal stethoscopes. The bell is designed to pick up lower frequency sounds, such as the diastolic murmur of mitral stenosis, and the diaphragm picks up most other sounds; however, on many modern stethoscopes the acoustic properties of the diaphragm are designed to change between those of a bell and those of a diaphragm depending on the pressure applied. It is important therefore to carefully read the manufacturer's instructions and become familiar with your stethoscope. The recordings on the CD were made using an electronic stethoscope, and these offer the ability to amplify the sounds. In day to day clinical activities however the authors use acoustic stethoscopes. It should also be noted that the longer the tube, the more likely it is for the sound to be dissipated: the standard length is recommended (approximately 50 cm). Remember that the best stethoscope cannot compete with background noise or an uncooperative patient!

Investigations

Electrocardiogram and chest radiograph

The electrocardiogram (ECG) and chest X-ray (CXR) give important information that may help to confirm a diagnosis or help to assess severity. We have therefore included a short note on possible ECG and CXR features, although detailed descriptions of the abnormalities are beyond the scope of this book. It will be noted through the book that while there may be specific ECG or CXR abnormalities, frequently these investigations may be normal even in the presence of significant disease.

Echocardiogram

Access to an echocardiogram is becoming more widespread in the United Kingdom, with general practitioners being able to access these services directly in some parts of the country. It is important to note however that the usefulness of an echocardiogram depends to a great extent on the skill and training of the operator, as well as the quality of the equipment and patient factors such as presence of subcutaneous fat, and their ability to move to, and hold a position to allow a satisfactory study. Before requesting an echocardiogram therefore, a clinician must be clear about the information that they wish to gain, understand the limitations of the examination, and be sure that this is the most appropriate investigation for these indications. Because of the widespread use of echocardiograms, a short sentence has been included about their assessment in each condition although detailed description is beyond the scope of this book.

Cardiac catheterization and magnetic resonance imaging

Full assessment of cardiac pathology increasingly includes the use of cardiac catheterization and cardiac magnetic resonance imaging and unlike echocardiography these investigations remain the province of specialist centres. These will not be covered in this book.

Learning point

- You only find what you look for.

▶ *Try for yourself*   **1.1 Normal heart sounds**

- Now listen to the recording of normal heart sounds on the CD. The recognition of abnormal heart sounds depends on the ability to appreciate, with certainty, the normal heart sounds, so use the following suggestions to ensure that you can with confidence identify the first and second heart sounds. Focus on S_1 while watching the systolic diastolic cursor (SDC) and note that S_1 coincides with the SDC landing on systole. When confident of timing of S_1, focus on S_2: note that S_2 coincides with the SDC landing on diastole.

- When you feel confident, minimize S_1 and see if you were right.

- When you have done this, reset, listen for a few cardiac cycles, again identify S_1 and S_2 then minimize S_2.

- Check that you had identified the correct sound.

- Finally listen again to the native recording. If you do not feel confident that you have identified S_1 and S_2, try maximizing each heart sound in turn until you can confidently identify the heart sounds in the native recording.

▶ *Try for yourself*   **1.2 Third heart sound**

- Now listen to the recording of the third heart sound on the CD and identify the first, second and third heart sounds. Use the suggestions to allow you to be confident of what you are hearing.

- First focus on S_1 while watching the SDC and note that S_1 coincides with the SDC landing on systole. When confident of the timing of S_1, focus on S_2. Note that S_2 coincides with the SDC landing on diastole. Next listen for the third heart sound in diastole.

- When you feel that you have identified this, minimize diastole. The third heart sound has now been eliminated.

- When you have listened for a few cardiac cycles reset to the native recording. If you could not appreciate the third heart sound before it should be easier now. This has been likened to a galloping horse.

- Repeat the previous two steps, minimizing then restoring diastole until you are confident that you can identify the third heart sound.

Aortic area (upper right sternal edge)

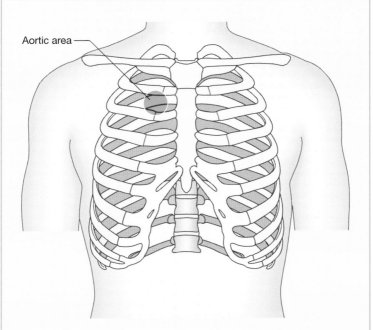

Aortic area

The aortic area is in the second right intercostal space

The murmurs best heard in this region are:
- Aortic stenosis
- Venous hum

Aortic stenosis

Anatomy

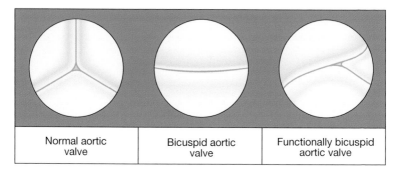

| Normal aortic valve | Bicuspid aortic valve | Functionally bicuspid aortic valve |

Fig. 2.1 *Aortic valve*

The aortic valve usually has three equal sized cusps. However abnormalities of the aortic valve are the most common congenital abnormality of the heart and are present in between 1 and 2 per cent of the population. The valve may be narrowed due to fusion between these cusps, or due to a valve with only two or even one cusp. Typically, in a stenotic trileaflet valve, the cusps are not of equal size. In congenital aortic stenosis, the valve annulus may also be small, and this is particularly true when the mitral valve is abnormal, or coarctation is also present (the Shone syndrome). A congenitally abnormal aortic valve is more likely to develop calcific stenosis in adult life, and this is more common if the cusps are of unequal size.

The aortic valve may also be narrowed due to thickening and myxomatous change in the valve. Don't forget that aortic regurgitation may co-exist in any patient with aortic stenosis (see Chapter 4).

The ascending aorta is often dilated in patients with bicuspid aortic valves or aortic stenosis. This is not post-stenotic dilatation because it does not reflect the severity of the stenosis, but is due to an abnormal aortic media.

History

In adults, aortic stenosis will usually be asymptomatic and detected because of the presence of a murmur, although patients may have angina, syncope on exercise, and rarely present with sudden death on exertion. Because calcific stenosis becomes more severe with time, a patient may not notice a gradual deterioration in his exercise tolerance. The condition is more common in men as bicuspid aortic valves are more common in men, with a male to female ratio of approximately four to one. The left ventricle will eventually fail and then the patient will develop breathlessness.

In neonates, critical aortic stenosis presents as a collapsed child with absent or very feeble pulses, respiratory distress and an enlarged liver. Outside the neonatal period, children will, like their adult counterparts, usually be asymptomatic and detected because of the presence of a murmur. An increase in the severity of the stenosis is not necessarily associated with a deterioration of symptoms. Syncope on exercise is a worrying symptom and may suggest the patient is at risk of sudden death.

Examination

In mild aortic stenosis, the general examination will be normal. In moderate to severe disease, the pulses may be of small volume and the pulse pressure narrow on blood pressure measurement. There may be a thrill in the suprasternal notch, or in more severe disease in the aortic area. The apex beat may be tapping in quality.

Patients with Turner's syndrome are more likely to have a bicuspid aortic valve and so features of this should be sought in girls with bicuspid aortic valves.

As already described, neonates may present collapsed with very poor pulses.

Heart sounds	S_1 normal S_2 normal, loud A2 in mild disease, softer as severity increases
Added sounds	Ejection click after S_1, loudest at the apex Fourth heart sound in severe stenosis Third heart sound in LV failure
Murmurs	Ejection systolic murmur in the aortic area radiating into the neck

ECG

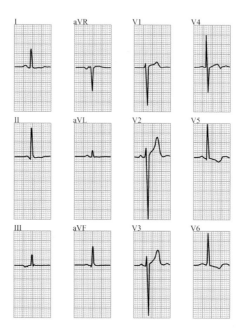

Fig. 2.2 *This patient has severe aortic stenosis. There is probable left ventricular hypertrophy on voltage criteria, with a deep S wave in lead V2. There is also left ventricular 'strain' pattern, with downward-sloping ST segment depression in leads V5 and V6*

In mild stenosis this will be normal. Unfortunately, in some patients increasing severity of stenosis is not reflected in the ECG which may remain normal. However usually increasing severity of stenosis will lead to left ventricular hypertrophy and then a left ventricular strain pattern on the ECG. These changes may be present on an exercise ECG when the resting ECG is normal, although performing exercise ECGs on patients with left ventricular outflow tract obstruction must be done with caution.

Neonates with critical aortic stenosis may show right ventricular hypertrophy due to pulmonary hypertension.

CXR

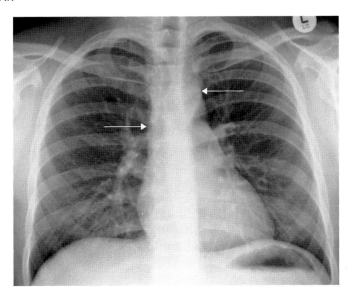

Fig. 2.3 Aortic stenosis. Note the prominent aortic shadow (arrows) indicating a dilated ascending aorta, common in this condition

This may well be normal, although post-stenotic dilatation of the ascending aorta may be seen and does not relate to severity of stenosis. Calcification may be visible in the valve cusps. Left ventricular hypertrophy may be visible in moderate to severe hypertrophy, and if the left ventricle fails, signs of raised left ventricular filling pressures and pulmonary oedema will be seen.

Echocardiogram

This will show the anatomy of the valve which may influence whether a surgical or catheter intervention is the first line of treatment. It will show the severity of stenosis and/or regurgitation and also allows assessment of left ventricular function.

Notes

The severity of aortic stenosis may progress throughout life. At the mildest end of the spectrum there may be only an ejection click from a bicuspid valve, not associated with stenosis or regurgitation. The click is difficult to appreciate in babies because of their relatively fast heart rate. The click will disappear if the valve becomes calcified. In patients with stenosis an ejection systolic murmur is heard, which is louder in more severe disease until the stenosis becomes severe and the cardiac output is compromised. The onset of left ventricular failure will further contribute to a reduction in the intensity of the murmur. The murmur of aortic stenosis is a crescendo/decrescendo murmur and the timing of maximal intensity becomes later as the stenosis becomes more severe, because left ventricular ejection becomes prolonged. With severe disease there may be reversed splitting of the second sound because of delay in the aortic component due to this prolongation of ventricular ejection. However, if the valve is very calcified and immobile, the aortic component of the second sound may be very soft or inaudible, so it may not be possible to hear this reversed splitting. The fourth heart sound occurs because of presystolic distension of the stiff, hypertrophied left ventricle. This implies significant disease, but is an unreliable sign of severity in patients older than 40 years. The third heart sound appears with left ventricular failure, and may add to the fourth heart sound to appear to be a mid-diastolic murmur.

Learning points

- The murmur of aortic stenosis is loudest in the aortic area but the click is loudest at the apex.
- An abnormal aortic valve may be associated with coarctation of the aorta.
- In very severe aortic stenosis, particularly when left ventricular failure supervenes, the murmur may be soft.

Summary

● Where is the murmur loudest?	→	Aortic area
● When does the murmur occur?	→	Systole
● What else could it be?	→	Still's murmur sometimes audible here but usually at the lower left sternal edge
● What makes it valvar aortic stenosis?	→	Quality of murmur, radiation into neck, click or thrill if present

Try for yourself **2.1 Valvar aortic stenosis (click)**

- Listen to the native recording which was made at the cardiac apex. There is only a very soft systolic murmur and the main feature of this recording is an ejection click. The click occurs almost immediately after S_1 and is very difficult to separate from it. Inexperienced auscultators often describe S_1 as being 'split', which is indeed what it sounds like.

- Maximize the click in order to make it clearer for you. Watch the SDC and time the heart sounds while trying to listen to the click.

- Next minimize the click and maximize S_1. The click has now gone and S_1 sounds single, loud and discrete.

- Next maximize the click and minimize S_1.

- Now S_1 has gone and only the click is present (which sounds remarkably like S_1).

- Finally leave the click on maximum and maximize S_1.

- Now both S_1 and the click are accentuated, and the 'double' sound is apparent.

- Repeat these four steps until you are sure that you can separately identify the first heart sound and the ejection click.

- Finally listen to the native recording and confirm that you can still identify the first heart sound and the aortic ejection click.

Try for yourself **2.2 Aortic stenosis (murmur)**

- This murmur was recorded in the aortic area where the murmur of aortic stenosis is loudest and the click is often inaudible. Listen to the soft first heart sound and the ejection systolic murmur which is clearly followed by S_2.

- When you have listened to the native murmur, try minimizing systole.

- This leaves only S_1 and S_2 audible. Sometimes it is easier to appreciate a murmur after it has been removed. Therefore next maximize systole.

- We have now enhanced the aortic stenosis murmur and made it much easier to hear.

- If necessary repeat the last two steps until you are confident that you are listening to the murmur.

- Finally replay the native murmur and appreciate the murmur as it was recorded.

Quiz

The following statements about aortic stenosis are true or false. Answer each one and then check the answers below to see if you are correct.

1. Abnormal aortic valves are more common in females than males.
2. Valvar aortic stenosis may lead to an aortic valve click.
3. The presence of a third heart sound indicates severe disease.
4. A dilated ascending aorta on CXR indicates severe aortic stenosis.
5. The murmur of aortic stenosis is a crescendo/decrescendo murmur.
6. A thrill associated with valvar aortic stenosis is best felt at the apex.
7. The second heart sound may be loud, soft or single in valvar aortic stenosis.
8. The ECG may be normal even with significant aortic stenosis.
9. Abnormal aortic valves may progress from predominant stenosis to predominant regurgitation.
10. Sudden death is a risk in important aortic stenosis.

Answers to quiz

1. False. The male:female ratio is about 4:1.
2. True. Although this may disappear if the valve becomes very immobile.
3. True, because this occurs in left ventricular failure.
4. False. Aortic root dilatation may occur in the presence of a bicuspid aortic valve without significant stenosis.
5. True. The later the peak of the murmur, the more severe the stenosis.
6. False. The apex beat may be tapping in quality, but the thrill is best felt at the upper right sternal edge and suprasternal notch. Occasionally in infants, the thrill may be to the left of the sternum, but moves to the right with growth.
7. True. A loud aortic component of the second sound occurs with a mobile valve and moderate stenosis. As the valve becomes less mobile, the second heart sound may become soft or single.
8. True. Although usually the ECG will show LVH with important aortic stenosis, it may be normal.
9. True. This may occur during childhood with growth. Occasionally valves which are predominantly regurgitant may progress with calcification and fibrosis to become predominantly stenotic.
10. True. This is particularly true on exercise.

Venous hum

Anatomy

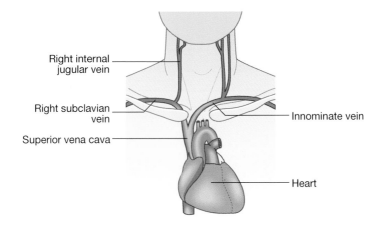

Right internal jugular vein

Right subclavian vein

Superior vena cava

Innominate vein

Heart

Fig. 2.4 *Great veins in the neck*

A venous hum is a common innocent murmur of childhood and, by definition, the cardiac anatomy is normal. The continuous noise originates from the great veins in the neck.

History

The patient will be asymptomatic. Venous hums are commonest from age 12 months to 6 years and so these murmurs are often detected on routine screening medical examinations. They may also be present in fit young adults, but also occur with a hyperdynamic circulation, such as in pregnancy, thyrotoxicosis or anaemia. Occasional patients are aware of the noise if it is loud, they experience it as pulsatile tinnitus.

Examination

General examination will be normal.

Heart sounds	S_1 normal
	S_2 normal
Added sounds	Nil
Murmurs	A continuous murmur, maximum above the clavicles just lateral to the sternocleidomastoid muscle, but often audible in the aortic and pulmonary areas

ECG
This will be normal.

CXR
This will be normal.

Echocardiogram
This will confirm a structurally normal heart.

Notes

Venous hums are low pitched continuous murmurs which are actually loudest above the clavicle, but are often heard below the clavicle, and are usually louder on the right than the left. They are accentuated by asking the subject to look over his or her shoulder and upwards, and are loudest when sitting and disappear when lying flat. They may be abolished by getting the subject to look in front and slightly downwards, or more reliably by pressure on the jugular vein, just lateral to the sternocleidomastoid muscle. They can be loud. As they may be heard below the clavicle they may be mistaken for a PDA, but they are lower pitched and the abolition by pressure confirms the true diagnosis.

Learning point
- A venous hum is a common innocent murmur in childhood.

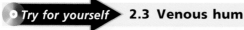

Try for yourself 2.3 Venous hum

- Now listen to the recording of a venous hum on the CD. Use these suggestions to ensure that you can hear the continuous murmur. At each step, ensure that you are clear what you are hearing before you move on.

- This recording was made below the clavicle on the left. There is a soft continuous murmur. The most difficult part of the murmur to appreciate is the diastolic component as initially most inexperienced auscultators interpret this as a systolic murmur. Try to appreciate its presence throughout the cardiac cycle while watching the SDC. The second heart sound in this example is loud. Try to hear that the murmur travels *through* S_2.

- When you feel that you are confident minimize diastole.

- You will now hear only the systolic component of this murmur and S_2 is the clearly defined end point. Having heard the isolated systolic component maximize diastole.

- The diastolic component is louder than before and so easier to hear. Listen until you are confident of its presence and if you are still unsure minimize systole (leaving diastole maximized).

- There is now a purely diastolic murmur. In this example you can still hear S_2, which now coincides with the beginning of the diastolic murmur (S_2 coincides with the SDC hitting diastole).

- Listen to the native murmur and be sure you appreciate its quality and timing. If you do not feel confident that you are hearing a continuous murmur, repeat the previous steps until you are confident.

Summary		
● Where is the murmur loudest?	→	Above the clavicle
● When does the murmur occur?	→	Throughout systole and diastole
● What else could it be?	→	A patent ductus arteriosus if loudest on the left
● What makes it a venous hum?	→	Variability with posture and pressure in the neck

Quiz

The following statements about venous hums are true or false. Try to answer them all and then check the answers below to see if you are correct.

1. Venous hums are common in childhood.
2. Venous hums are systolic.
3. Venous hums are louder on lying flat.
4. A venous hum may be mistaken for a PDA.
5. Venous hums are usually louder on the left.
6. A venous hum is obliterated by pressing on the ipsilateral internal jugular vein.
7. A venous hum may be more prominent during a febrile illness.
8. A venous hum may present as tinnitus.
9. Venous hums may be heard over the left lung.
10. The cause of a venous hum may be seen on echocardiography.

Answers to quiz

1. True. They are common in children and young adults.
2. False, they are continuous, through systole and diastole.
3. False. They are loudest when sitting and may disappear on lying flat.
4. True, although generally they are lower pitched than PDA murmurs.
5. False, they are usually louder on the right.
6. True, which confirms the diagnosis.
7. True, and also during pregnancy or in the presence of anaemia.
8. True, this has been described.
9. False. A loud PDA murmur is sometimes heard at the back.
10. False. Although it is postulated that the noise originates from the internal jugular vein being distorted by the spinous process of a vertebra this is not proven.

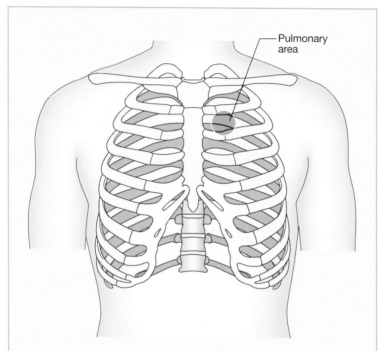

Pulmonary area

The pulmonary area is in the second left intercostal space

The auscultatory abnormalities best heard in this region are:

- Atrial septal defect
- Pulmonary stenosis
- Innocent pulmonary flow
- Patent ductus arteriosus
- Loud second heart sound

Atrial septal defect

Anatomy

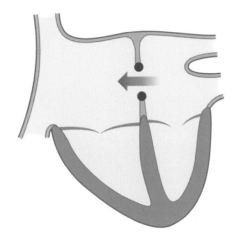

Fig. 3.1 *Atrial septal defect*

An atrial septal defect (ASD) is a hole in the atrial septum. Because the right atrial pressure is, for most of the time, lower than the left atrial pressure, this allows blood to flow from left atrium to right atrium. This leads to an increase in size (dilatation) of the right atrium and ventricle and increased blood flow to the lungs.

At times, such as after straining (for example during childbirth), the right atrial pressure exceeds the left atrial pressure, which causes the flow to be right to left across the ASD.

Most commonly the hole is in the region of the normal fetal structure, the fossa ovalis (secundum ASD). The hole may be at the atrioventricular valve junction and is then associated with abnormal atrioventricular valves and mitral regurgitation (primum ASD, partial/incomplete atrioventricular septal defect). The hole may be at the junction of the superior vena cava or inferior vena cava with the right atrium (sinus venosus ASD), and is then associated with partial anomalous pulmonary venous drainage. *However, the signs and symptoms in each case are identical.*

History

ASDs are often asymptomatic until complications arise in adulthood; however, they may be associated with chestiness and failure to thrive in childhood.

Complications arise from the physiological changes detailed above and are thus:

1. atrial or ventricular arrhythmias due to the enlarged right heart;
2. frequent chest infections and eventually pulmonary hypertension due to increased pulmonary blood flow;
3. and stroke due to paradoxical embolism.

Examination

As always, look for signs of any recognizable syndrome. Down's syndrome is particularly associated with ostium primum ASDs. Feel for right ventricular heave (from dilated right heart or pulmonary hypertension) and a palpable second heart sound (only in pulmonary hypertension).

Heart sounds	S_1, normal
	S_2, widely split
Added sounds	*Nil*
Murmurs	*Systole: ejection systolic murmur, often transmitted to the back*
	Diastole: usually silent or soft tricuspid flow murmur

ECG

The ECG may be normal. It may show a rightward axis, prolonged PR interval and incomplete right bundle branch block. Ostium primum defects and some sinus venosus defects are associated with a superior axis. If there is pulmonary hypertension then voltage criteria for right ventricular hypertrophy may be satisfied.

CXR

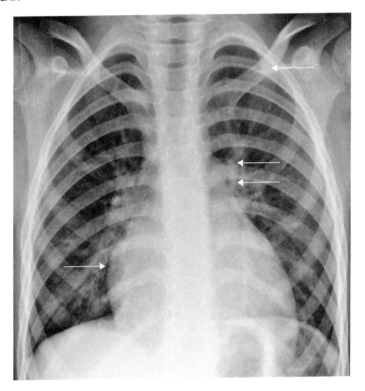

Fig. 3.2 *Atrial septal defect. This shows a large heart, particularly the right atrium (single arrow), right ventricle and central pulmonary arteries (double arrows). The lung fields will appear plethoric, although if pulmonary hypertension develops, there will be peripheral pruning of the vessels*

This shows a large heart, particularly the right atrium, right ventricle and central pulmonary arteries. The lung fields will appear plethoric, although if pulmonary hypertension develops there will be peripheral pruning of the vessels.

Echocardiography

This will confirm the diagnosis of an ASD, and allow an assessment of the anatomy to see whether it is suitable for catheter device closure or surgery. An assessment of pulmonary hypertension can be made, as this may preclude closure. The presence of associated lesions, such as pulmonary stenosis will also be assessed.

Notes

ASDs vary in size from only a few millimetres to almost complete absence of the septum. There is therefore a range of haemodynamics, which is mirrored by the auscultatory findings. Classical teaching describes *wide fixed splitting* and indeed this is usually the case in *large* defects. In smaller defects, the second sound may be more narrowly split and somewhat variable, and sometimes difficult to differentiate from normal splitting. With the establishment of pulmonary hypertension the pulmonary component will become accentuated and the splitting reduced. The intensity of the pulmonary ejection murmur varies and, somewhat surprisingly, does not always correlate with defect size; however, the presence of a tricuspid diastolic murmur does suggest heavy flow through a large defect.

Learning points

- The classic signs of an ASD are not found if pulmonary hypertension supervenes
- Wide fixed splitting occurs in large defects
- Smaller ASDs may be associated with narrower splitting, which may be somewhat variable

Summary

• Where is the murmur loudest?	→ Pulmonary area
• When does the murmur occur?	→ Mid systole
• What else could it be?	→ Valvar pulmonary stenosis or innocent pulmonary flow murmur
• What makes it an ASD?	→ Presence of wide splitting of second sound

Try for yourself **3.1 Atrial septal defect**

- Now listen to the recording of an atrial septal defect on the CD. Use these suggestions to ensure that you can hear the splitting of the second heart sound and the soft pulmonary flow murmur. At each step, ensure that you are clear what you are hearing before you move on.

- An atrial septal defect may be one of the most difficult diagnoses to make clinically. The murmur is soft and systolic and the main clue to the underlying aetiology is the wide fixed splitting of the second heart sound. As you listen, concentrate on the second heart sound. Splitting of the second sound, even when it is wide, is subtle. Note that S_2 occurs as the SDC hits diastole. Splitting may be likened to tapping the middle (first) and index (second) fingers of your right hand *almost* simultaneously onto a wooden table.

- When you have listened to the native murmur, minimize systole.

- This eliminates the systolic murmur and allows you to focus on S_2. Try to appreciate the splitting and don't worry, it is not that obvious. When you have listened for a few cycles, maximize the S_2 split.

- Listen carefully and focus on S_2. The systolic murmur is quiet and we have widened the splitting, making it easier to appreciate. Listen until you feel you can appreciate the splitting. When you feel that you can hear the enhanced splitting, reset then maximize the systolic murmur.

- Listen carefully. The murmur is soft and quite short but is now louder and more easily appreciated.

- Finally listen to the native recording and be sure you appreciate the splitting of S_2 as well as the soft systolic murmur. Repeat the steps above, increasing and decreasing the intensity of the murmur and increasing and decreasing the split of S_2 until you are confident of the heart sounds audible in a patient with an ASD.

Quiz

The following statements are true or false. Cover the answers to test your understanding.

1. The murmur associated with an atrial septal defect is related to turbulent flow across the atrial communication.
2. In an atrial septal defect there is always fixed splitting of the second sound.
3. In general, the wider the splitting of the second sound the greater the left to right shunt across the atrial septal defect.
4. The presence of a tricuspid diastolic murmur associated with an atrial septal defect usually means that intervention is indicated.
5. Pulmonary hypertension is a common early complication of atrial septal defects.
6. The presence of right ventricular hypertrophy on the ECG should alert you to the possibility of pulmonary hypertension.
7. A superior axis on the ECG is usual in a secundum atrial septal defect.
8. Patients with a primum atrial septal defect often present earlier than those with a secundum ASD.
9. A pulmonary diastolic murmur may occur with the onset of pulmonary hypertension.
10. On chest radiograph, a prominent aorta may reflect a large shunt.

Answers to quiz

1. False. The murmur comes from increased flow across the pulmonary outflow tract.
2. False. The splitting of the second sound is widened in an atrial septal defect but it may still be variable, particularly in smaller defects.
3. True. With larger defects there is more flow and the split becomes wider.
4. True. Tricuspid diastolic murmurs tend to be associated with larger defects.
5. False. Pulmonary hypertension due to an atrial septal defect does not tend to occur until the fourth or fifth decade of life, and may not be present even in older patients. Patients with primary pulmonary hypertension may maintain an atrial communication as this helps cardiac output.

6. True. There may be generous right ventricular voltages on ECG due to right ventricular dilatation, but in general if there is right ventricular hypertrophy then pulmonary hypertension needs to be suspected.

7. False. A superior axis is more typical of a primum ASD (partial atrioventricular septal defect).

8. True. Primum atrial septal defect (partial atrioventricular septal defect) is commonly associated with regurgitation of the left or right atrioventricular valves, leading to murmurs that are more easily heard than those of a simple secundum atrial septal defect. Primum atrial septal defect is also more common in patients with trisomy 21 and therefore may be detected as the result of routine screening.

9. True. With elevated diastolic pulmonary artery pressure, the pulmonary valve may become regurgitant.

10. False. The pulmonary artery may appear prominent in the setting of a large shunt, and the ascending aorta may be relatively inconspicuous.

Valvar pulmonary stenosis

Anatomy

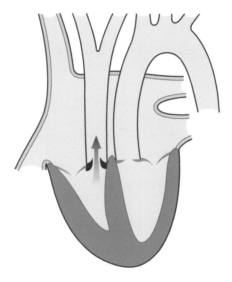

Fig. 3.3 *Valvar pulmonary stenosis*

Valvar pulmonary stenosis is narrowing at the level of the pulmonary valve. It may be due to fusion of the commissures of a bicuspid or tricuspid valve, or to a thickened myxomatous valve with limited movement. A very thickened dysplastic valve is more common in pulmonary stenosis associated with a syndrome (such as Noonan syndrome). The narrow valve leads to turbulent blood flow. The right ventricular pressure rises with increasing severity of stenosis in order to maintain blood flow to the lungs. As the stenosis becomes more severe, however, the right ventricle will be unable to overcome the obstruction and will fail.

History

Mild pulmonary stenosis is asymptomatic. It is detected because of the presence of a typical murmur, which is louder at times of high cardiac output, such as in a febrile illness or during pregnancy. Gradients across the pulmonary valve of less than 40 mmHg are unlikely to progress.

Moderate to severe pulmonary stenosis may also be asymptomatic, but may present with breathlessness and fatigue, particularly on exercise, due to the inability of the right ventricle to increase its output in the face of the limiting obstruction.

In the neonatal period, pulmonary stenosis may be critical, in which the blood returning to the right heart cannot be ejected through the pulmonary valve because of the severity of the obstruction. This may be associated with an anatomically small right ventricle. The baby will be well (although cyanosed) while the ductus arteriosus is patent, and if the foramen ovale allows right to left shunting of blood to bypass the right ventricle, but will become severely unwell when the duct closes.

Examination

As always, look for signs of any recognizable syndrome. Noonan syndrome is particularly associated with pulmonary stenosis. General examination will usually be otherwise normal, although in severe pulmonary stenosis with right ventricular failure there may be a raised jugular venous pressure, ankle oedema and hepatomegaly. In critical pulmonary stenosis the baby will appear cyanosed and may be breathless and have a poor systemic cardiac output. In severe pulmonary stenosis there may be a right ventricular heave and a thrill palpable in the pulmonary area.

Heart sounds	S_1, normal
	S_2, normal
Added sounds	*Systolic ejection click after first heart sound*
Murmurs	*Systole: ejection systolic murmur radiating through to back*
	Diastole: usually nil

ECG

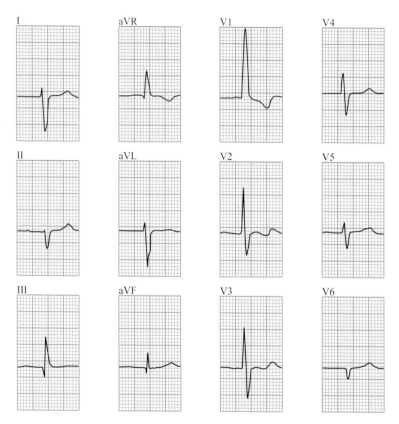

Fig. 3.4 *This infant presented with severe pulmonary valve stenosis. Unusually, the P waves are very low voltage but there is sinus rhythm with the P wave most obvious in lead II. Note that there is prolongation of the PR interval (first degree heart block, PR interval approximately 240 ms). There is right axis deviation (QRS axis approximately 145 degrees), a common finding in right ventricular hypertrophy. There are voltage criteria for severe right ventricular hypertrophy with a pure R wave in lead V1 and a pure S wave in lead V6*

This will be normal in mild to moderate pulmonary stenosis, but will show right ventricular hypertrophy with right ventricular strain in severe cases. In Noonan syndrome there may be a superior axis. In neonates with critical pulmonary stenosis and a small right ventricle there may be an inappropriate lack of right ventricular forces present on the neonatal ECG.

CXR

This will usually be normal, although the main pulmonary artery may be prominent due to post-stenotic dilatation, which is not an indication of severity. In more severe pulmonary stenosis there will be right ventricular hypertrophy with an upturned cardiac apex, and cardiomegaly once the right ventricle has failed. In the neonate with critical pulmonary stenosis there will be pulmonary oligaemia, although the cardiac contour may be quite normal.

Echocardiogram

The echocardiogram will demonstrate the pulmonary stenosis and allow an assessment of the severity of the obstruction. The function of the right ventricle will also be assessed, as well as a search made for associated lesions such as atrial communications.

Notes

There may be an audible valve click. With increasing severity the click moves closer towards the first heart sound, so in very severe stenosis the click may become inaudible. There will be a systolic murmur that radiates through to the back. With increasing severity the murmur will become louder and may become associated with a thrill; however, with even more severe disease as the ventricle fails and as the cardiac output of the right ventricle falls, the murmur will become quieter again.

Learning point
• Valvar pulmonary stenosis may be part of complex congenital heart disease.

Summary		
• Where is the murmur loudest?	→	Pulmonary area
• When does the murmur occur?	→	Mid systole
• What else could it be?	→	ASD or innocent pulmonary flow murmur
• What makes it valvar pulmonary stenosis?	→	Presence of valve click Absense of wide splitting of second sound

▶ *Try for yourself*   3.2 Valvar pulmonary stenosis

- Now listen to the recording of a valvar pulmonary stenosis on the CD. Use these suggestions to ensure that you can hear the valvar click and the pulmonary stenosis murmur. At each step, ensure that you are clear what you are hearing before you move on.

- This murmur was recorded in the pulmonary area. As you listen to the native recording first listen to the systolic murmur then try to hear the ejection click just after the first heart sound. When you feel that you have identified both sounds you can manipulate the heart sounds to be sure that you are right.

- First minimize systole.

- Having eliminated the systolic murmur you can focus on the heart sounds. S_1 coincides with the SDC hitting systole. Immediately after S_1 is an ejection click. It is discrete and crisp and it is often mistaken for S_1 itself. When you feel that you have identified this, minimize S_1.

- Listen and note that most of the time there is no S_1, and the click is the first sound.

- When you feel confident that you can hear the click, maximize S_1.

- You should now be more confident that you can hear two separate sounds, S_1 followed by the ejection click.

- Finally reset and listen to the native murmur and confirm in order S_1, ejection click, ejection systolic murmur and S_2. Use this case to learn to separate the click from S_1.

Quiz

The following statements are true or false. Cover the answers to test your understanding;

1. In pulmonary stenosis, the louder the murmur, the worse the narrowing.
2. Even mild pulmonary stenosis usually leads to symptoms.
3. Neonates with critical pulmonary stenosis are cyanosed.
4. A pulmonary valve click may occur without a murmur.
5. Post stenotic dilatation of the pulmonary artery on chest radiograph always indicates severe disease.
6. The murmur of pulmonary stenosis is best heard in the pulmonary area.
7. Pulmonary stenosis murmurs are diastolic.
8. A pulmonary stenosis murmur may be louder during pregnancy.
9. Pulmonary stenosis may be present despite a normal ECG and CXR.
10. Mild pulmonary stenosis always requires invasive treatment.

Answers to quiz

1. False. Although this is true up to a point, with very severe stenosis the cardiac output falls and the murmur becomes quieter.
2. False. Mild pulmonary stenosis is usually asymptomatic.
3. True. This is due to decreased pulmonary blood flow and right to left shunting at atrial level.
4. True. Bicuspid or mildly abnormal valves may click but not be significantly narrow and so not generate a murmur.
5. False. Severe stenosis may be associated with small pulmonary arteries and an abnormal valve may be associated with dilatation of the pulmonary artery without stenosis.
6. True. The position of the murmur gives a clue to the diagnosis.
7. False. The stenosis murmur is systolic. A diastolic murmur may come from associated pulmonary regurgitation.
8. True. Any condition which increases the cardiac output, such as pregnancy, may result in a louder murmur.
9. True. Even with moderate stenosis these investigations may be normal.
10. False. Mild pulmonary stenosis is well tolerated and may never progress.

Innocent pulmonary flow murmur

Anatomy

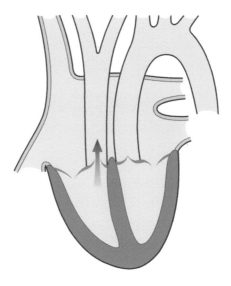

Fig. 3.5 *Innocent pulmonary flow murmur*

By definition the cardiac anatomy is normal in any innocent murmur. Pulmonary flow murmurs are, however, thought to arise from the right ventricular outflow tract.

History

These patients have structurally and functionally normal hearts, and therefore cannot have any cardiac symptoms. Innocent murmurs are very common in childhood and therefore by chance some children with symptoms such as chest pain, which are actually non-cardiac in origin, will have co-existing innocent murmurs.

Examination

The cardiovascular examination will be normal apart from the murmur. The presence of dysmorphic features makes structural heart disease more likely, but because innocent murmurs are common in childhood there will by chance be some of these patients who have innocent murmurs.

Heart sounds	S_1, normal
	S_2, normal
Added sounds	Nil
Murmurs	Systole: ejection systolic murmur
	Diastole: nil

ECG
This will be normal.

CXR
This will be normal.

Echocardiogram
This will confirm a structurally normal heart.

Notes

Innocent pulmonary flow murmurs are common, particularly in childhood, but also in young adults, especially in hyperdynamic states such as pregnancy. They do not radiate to the back.

Learning point

- The distinction between an innocent pulmonary flow murmur and an ASD depends upon assessment of the splitting of the second heart sound and may be very difficult.

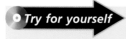

Try for yourself ➤ **3.3 Innocent pulmonary flow murmur**

- Now listen to the recording of an innocent pulmonary flow murmur on the CD. Use these suggestions to ensure that you can hear the murmur and compare it in your mind to the murmurs associated with valvar pulmonary stenosis and atrial septal defect. At each step, ensure that you are clear what you are hearing before you move on.

- As you listen to the native murmur, watch the SDC and note that the murmur coincides with it hitting systole and is very soft (1/6 in intensity). Try to appreciate S_1 and S_2, which are clearly and discretely audible. The main diagnostic feature of this murmur is that it is soft and does not radiate. When you have listened to the native murmur maximize systole.

- This has made the murmur louder and, if you could not hear it before, it should be more apparent now. Watch the SDC and time the two heart sounds. When you feel confident that you can hear the murmur, minimize systole. This has removed the murmur.

- Try making the murmur louder and quieter until you are confident that you can hear the pulmonary flow murmur.

Summary

● Where is the murmur loudest?	➤	Pulmonary area
● When does the murmur occur?	➤	Mid systole
● What else could it be?	➤	ASD or valvular pulmonary stenosis
● What makes it innocent pulmonary flow murmur?	➤	Normal second sound and lack of radiation of murmur

Quiz

The following statements about innocent pulmonary flow murmurs are true or false. Answer each one and then check the answers below to see if you are correct.

1. If a child has any symptoms a murmur cannot be innocent.
2. Distinguishing between an innocent pulmonary flow murmur and an ASD on auscultation depends upon the second heart sound.
3. ECG and chest radiograph will be normal in an innocent murmur.
4. An innocent pulmonary flow murmur may be louder during a febrile illness.
5. Innocent pulmonary flow murmurs frequently radiate to the back.
6. Innocent pulmonary flow murmurs are loudest at the lower left sternal edge.
7. Innocent pulmonary flow murmurs are often associated with an ejection click.
8. Innocent pulmonary flow murmurs are systolic.
9. Innocent pulmonary flow murmurs are associated with a right ventricular heave.
10. Innocent pulmonary flow murmurs can occur in adults.

Answers to quiz

1. False. Because innocent murmurs are so common in childhood, some children with non-cardiac symptoms will have an incidental unrelated murmur.
2. True. The presence of wide splitting indicates an ASD. This can be a difficult sign to elicit.
3. True, but they may also be normal in the presence of mild to moderate pulmonary stenosis.
4. True, indeed in some children they may not be present when the child is well.
5. False. A murmur that radiates to the back is almost always pathological.
6. False. They are loudest in the pulmonary area.
7. False. An ejection click would indicate the presence of an abnormal pulmonary valve.
8. True.
9. False. The presence of a thrill or heave indicates a pathological murmur.
10. True.

Patent ductus arteriosus

Anatomy

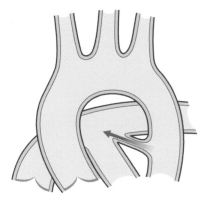

Fig. 3.6 *Patent ductus arteriosus*

The ductus arteriosus is a normal fetal structure that connects the main pulmonary artery with the descending aorta. It may remain patent after birth, particularly in babies born prematurely, sick newborns from any cause, and in the presence of structural heart disease. There is also a familial form of patent ductus arteriosus (PDA).

History

Large ducts may be associated with failure to thrive, and breathlessness or chestiness in childhood. Irreversible pulmonary hypertension may occur in childhood if the duct is large.

Examination

In large ducts the pulses will be full volume, with a wide pulse pressure (difference between systolic and diastolic blood pressure). The cardiac impulse will be active and the apex beat may be displaced towards the axilla due to enlargement of the left ventricle. The liver may enlarge and breathlessness can be prominent, particularly in young babies. On auscultation there will be a continuous murmur audible throughout systole and into diastole. Note that continuous murmurs extend through the second sound but are not necessarily present throughout the whole cardiac cycle. The patent ductus murmur is loudest under the left clavicle, but may be audible throughout the precordium and posteriorly on the left. In large ducts there may be a mitral diastolic flow murmur audible at the apex.

Heart sounds	S_1, normal S_2, normal
Added sounds	Nil
Murmurs	Systole: continuous murmur, extending through second heart sound Diastole: continuous murmur, although may be quiet in late diastole

ECG

This will be normal in the presence of a small duct. Large ducts with large left-to-right shunts may show left ventricular volume overload with left ventricular hypertrophy on voltage criteria or generous biventricular voltages. If pulmonary hypertension develops there will be right ventricular hypertrophy, with right ventricular strain as the severity increases.

CXR

This will also be normal in small ducts. In the presence of a larger duct, the heart will enlarge (mainly the left ventricular contour) with pulmonary plethora and an enlarged pulmonary artery. With pulmonary hypertension, there will be an enlarged heart (mainly the right ventricle) with large central pulmonary arteries but peripheral pruning.

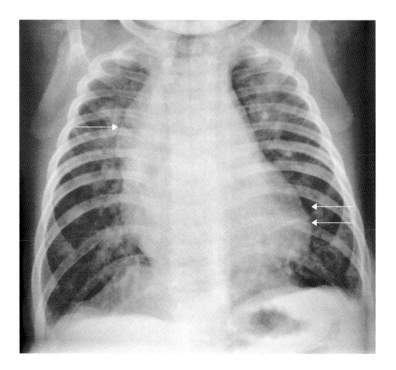

Fig. 3.7 *This baby has a large patent ductus arteriosus. The thymus is prominent (arrow) and normal. There is cardiomegaly (with an LV contour, double arrow) and plethora because of the left-to-right shunt. The chest is hyperinflated*

Echocardiography

This will confirm the presence of a patent ductus arteriosus. An assessment of suitability for closure via a cardiac catheter can be made, including estimating the pulmonary artery pressure. Careful assessment of all the cardiac anatomy is mandatory to ensure that there are no associated lesions, such as pulmonary stenosis or coarctation of the aorta.

Notes

In large ducts there may be signs of 'heart failure', with hepatomegaly, failure to thrive and breathlessness. A wide pulse pressure, active precordium and mitral flow murmur are also signs of a large left-to-right shunt. If pulmonary hypertension supervenes, the continuous murmur will become quieter and shorter, and the second sound louder. With severe pulmonary hypertension, there will be a right ventricular heave, a loud and palpable second heart sound and pulmonary regurgitation may develop. Rarely, with reversal of the shunt through the duct there may be differential cyanosis and clubbing affecting the toes but not the fingers.

Learning point

- The murmur of a PDA may be mistaken for a venous hum.

Summary

• Where is the murmur loudest? ➔	Upper left sternal edge, under the clavicle
• When does the murmur occur? ➔	Throughout systole into diastole
• What else could it be? ➔	A venous hum is continuous but low pitched, louder in the neck and altered by pressure in the anterior triangle
• What makes it a PDA? ➔	Continuous high pitched murmur in pulmonary area

> **Try for yourself** **3.4 Patent ductus arteriosus**

- Now listen to the recording of a patent ductus arteriosus on the CD. Use these suggestions to ensure that you can hear the murmur. At each step, ensure that you are clear what you are hearing before you move on.

- As you listen to the recording try to appreciate a continuous murmur which is described as machinery and is typical of a PDA. The murmur is loudest in the left infraclavicular region, where this recording was made. Time the murmur with the SDC. The systolic component is well appreciated. Try to hear the murmur continuing over the second heart sound into diastole, keeping focused on the SDC. To help to appreciate the continuous nature of the murmur, minimize diastole.

- S_1 and S_2 are quite soft. Listen to the systolic murmur for a few cycles and then concentrate on diastole after S_2. Note that there is now no sound there. Watch the SDC while listening. When you are happy with this maximize diastole.

- You have now reintroduced the diastolic component of the murmur and increased its volume. Listen to the systolic murmur and notice how it extends over the second heart sound. This is the diastolic component of the PDA murmur and the systolic and diastolic components run into each other, i.e. the murmur is continuous. Listen carefully for as long as it takes to appreciate fully this part of the murmur. If you are still having difficulty differentiating the systolic component from the diastolic, then minimize systole.

- Now that there is no systolic murmur only the diastolic component remains. When you have listened for a few cycles maximize systole.

- Now both the systolic and diastolic components are set at maximum intensity. Listen until you are confident that you are clearly separating the two components.

- Listen finally to the native murmur and again time with the SDC. You should now be able to appreciate that the murmur runs through systole and diastole.

Quiz

The following statements are true or false. Cover the answers to test your understanding.

1. A PDA murmur is typically described as a machinery murmur.
2. The murmur of a PDA is best heard under the left clavicle.
3. A PDA murmur may become shorter with time.
4. Continuous murmurs are there throughout the whole cardiac cycle.
5. A low diastolic blood pressure may be a sign of a patent ductus arteriosus.
6. Patent arterial ducts are common in babies born prematurely.
7. There may be a mitral diastolic murmur associated with a tiny duct.
8. The presence of a patent ductus arteriosus is not associated with an increased risk of endocarditis.
9. A large patent ductus arteriosus may have no murmur.
10. A patent ductus arteriosus may be found with complex congenital heart disease.

Answers to quiz

1. True. This only applies to moderate sized ducts with a large pressure drop across them. It is not usual in neonates or with PHT.
2. True. It may radiate widely over the chest.
3. True. If PHT develops, the murmur becomes shorter and quieter.
4. False. Continuous murmurs cross the second heart sound but are not present for the whole of the cardiac cycle.
5. True. The lower resistance of the pulmonary bed leads to a shunting in diastole and a low diastolic blood pressure.
6. True. These ducts may close spontaneously with time, but may require active treatment if the baby is symptomatic.
7. False. The presence of a mitral diastolic murmur indicates a heavy left-to-right shunt and so a medium or large duct.
8. False. An audible patent ductus arteriosus has one of the highest rates of endocarditis and this is an indication for closing these ducts.
9. True. The murmur comes from turbulent flow across the duct so if there is no restriction to flow, and particularly in neonates with elevated pulmonary artery pressure, there may be no murmur.
10. True. A patent duct may be useful in the setting of complex congenital heart disease and may be maintained with prostin.

Loud second heart sound

The second sound may be loud because the pulmonary component is loud, for example in pulmonary hypertension, or it may be loud because of an abnormal position of the aorta. This occurs when the aorta is shifted towards the sternum in conditions such as transposition of the great arteries or tetralogy of Fallot. In some conditions where the heart functions as if it had a single ventricle the aorta may be anterior.

The history and other examination findings associated with a loud second heart sound will depend upon its underlying cause.

● Try for yourself   3.5 Loud second heart sound

- Now listen to the recording of a loud second heart sound on the CD. Use these suggestions to ensure that you can appreciate the loud second sound. At each step, ensure that you are clear what you are hearing before you move on.

- This murmur was recorded in the pulmonary area in a patient with pulmonary hypertension. Focus on S_1 while watching the SDC and note that S_1 coincides with the SDC landing on systole. When confident of the timing of S_1, focus on S_2. Note that S_2 coincides with SDC landing on diastole. S_2 is loud and crisp. In order to appreciate the loud second sound, further maximize S_2.

- The S_2 is now very loud. When you are confident of the timing of S_2, minimize S_2.

- Note the phonocardiogram now without an S_2. Sometimes removing the sound makes it easier to appreciate when it returns.

- Finally listen again to the native recording and be sure that you are confident of the timing of S_1 and S_2 and the increased intensity of S_2.

Mid left sternal edge

4

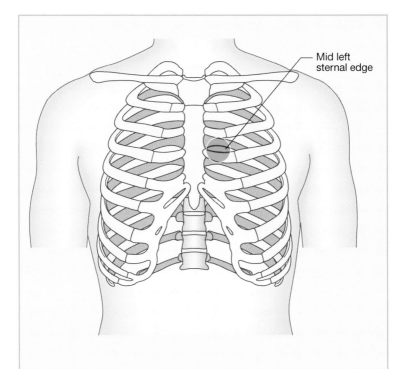

Mid left
sternal edge

The auscultatory abnormalities best heard in this region are:
- Aortic regurgitation
- Subvalvar pulmonary stenosis
- Pulmonary regurgitation
- Splitting of the second sound in right bundle branch block

Aortic regurgitation

Anatomy

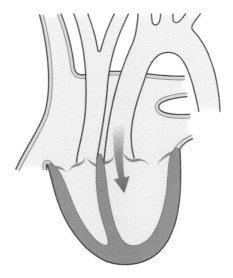

Fig. 4.1 *Aortic regurgitation*

Aortic regurgitation may be the predominant lesion in a congenitally bicuspid aortic valve, or it may occur following balloon or surgical valvotomy for aortic stenosis. It may also develop with an anatomically normal aortic valve in the presence of aortic root dilatation or following damage to a previously normal valve due to endocarditis or rheumatic fever.

History

Bicuspid aortic valves are more common in men and boys, and therefore so is aortic regurgitation. Aortic regurgitation may cause shortness of breath on exertion, but if the onset is gradual the patient may be asymptomatic even in the presence of severe aortic incompetence.

Examination

There will be no abnormal cardiac physical signs in mild aortic regurgitation other than the murmur. As severity increases there may be nailbed capillary pulsation, full volume pulses, a wide pulse pressure, a prominent left ventricular impulse and a displaced cardiac apex. If the onset is acute, severe aortic regurgitation will lead to a low cardiac output so the usual physical signs may be absent.

Heart sounds	S_1, normal
	S_2, aortic component diminished
Added sounds	Nil, ejection click, S_3
Murmurs	Early diastolic decrescendo murmur

ECG

This may be normal or show voltage criteria for left ventricular hypertrophy. Repolarization changes are not uncommon in aortic regurgitation.

CXR

In mild aortic regurgitation the CXR may be normal. The cardiac silhouette may be enlarged with a left ventricular contour. The ascending aorta may be prominent. In acute severe aortic regurgitation there may be pulmonary oedema with minimal cardiomegaly.

Echocardiography

This will reveal the cause of the regurgitation (for example dilated aortic root, prolapsing valve cusp or hole in cusp from endocarditis). The severity can also be assessed, both by measuring the size of the left ventricle, and using colour flow mapping.

Notes

A soft aortic systolic ejection murmur in aortic regurgitation can be present because of increased left ventricular stroke volume. In chronic aortic regurgitation the length and intensity of the murmur relate to the degree of aortic regurgitation. Furthermore, the more severe the regurgitation, the lower the pitch of the murmur. Important aortic regurgitation may be associated with a low pitched mid-diastolic murmur at the apex due to early partial closure of the mitral valve caused by the regurgitant jet (the Austin Flint murmur). In acute severe aortic regurgitation there may be a paucity of auscultatory findings.

Learning points

- The murmur of aortic regurgitation is decrescendo early diastolic
- The murmur is accentuated by leaning forward and breathing out
- Pitch as well as length and intensity relate to severity of regurgitation
- A murmur may be absent in acute severe aortic regurgitation

Summary

● Where is the murmur loudest?	→	Mid left sternal edge
● When does the murmur occur?	→	Diastole
● What else could it be?	→	Pulmonary regurgitation in the presence of pulmonary hypertension
● What makes it an aortic regurgitation murmur?	→	Pitch and position of the murmur and diastolic timing

Try for yourself **4.1 Aortic regurgitation**

- Now listen to the recording of aortic regurgitation on the CD. Use these suggestions to ensure that you can hear the diastolic murmur. At each step, ensure that you are clear what you are hearing before you move on.

- This recording was made at the lower left sternal edge in a patient without a significant systolic murmur.

- Start the recording and listen to the early diastolic murmur. This is often described as blowing.

- Use the SDC to be clear that you can hear the murmur in diastole. The inexperienced auscultator often mistimes this murmur as systolic or, alternatively, does not hear it at all. Now minimize diastole to eliminate the diastolic component and ensure that you are listening to the correct sound.

- There is now a soft S_1 and a louder S_2. Listen to this for a few cycles and watch the SDC. Note now that there is a clear gap after S_2 where there is silence in diastole. When you are confident with this maximize diastole.

- Focus on the SDC and note S_1 and S_2. The diastolic murmur is now loud and immediately follows S_2 and occurs when the SDC hits diastole. Repeat the last two steps, minimizing and maximizing diastole until you are confident that you have identified the aortic regurgitation murmur.

- Finally, listen again to the native murmur and time the murmur against the SDC. You should now be able to appreciate the diastolic murmur as it was recorded.

Quiz

The following statements are true or false. Cover the answers to test your understanding.

1. Severe aortic regurgitation is always associated with a loud murmur.
2. Aortic regurgitation may occur with a normal aortic valve.
3. Aortic regurgitation may occur after treatment of aortic stenosis.
4. Aortic regurgitation may occur because of bacterial endocarditis.
5. The murmur of aortic regurgitation is systolic.
6. A wide pulse pressure is a sign of chronic important aortic regurgitation.
7. If the apex beat is in the normal position, there cannot be AR.
8. Aortic regurgitation shows a female preponderance.
9. Aortic regurgitation may be present in Marfan's syndrome.
10. Chronic aortic regurgitation is always symptomatic.

Answers to quiz

1. False. In acute AR, there may be low cardiac output and no murmur.
2. True. If there is aortic root dilatation, for example in Marfan's syndrome, a normal aortic valve may leak.
3. True. AR may occur after surgical or balloon valvotomy.
4. True. A congenitally abnormal aortic valve is more likely to develop endocarditis. The resulting AR may be acute and severe.
5. False. The murmur of AR is diastolic, although there may be a systolic murmur due to the increase in cardiac output.
6. True. The regurgitation in diastole leads to a drop in diastolic pressure. This adaptation is not present in acute aortic regurgitation.
7. False. In mild AR the apex beat may be normal. In acute severe AR (such as associated with endocarditis) the left ventricle may be unable to dilate and the cardiac output falls.
8. False. There is a male preponderance because congenital abnormalities of the aortic valve are more common in males.
9. True. The aortic dilatation of Marfan's syndrome may lead to leakage through an anatomically normal valve.
10. False. Mild to moderate AR may be present for many years before symptoms develop.

Subvalvar pulmonary stenosis

Anatomy

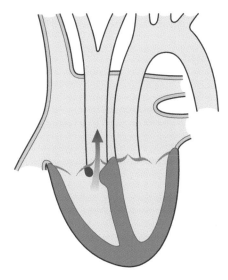

Fig. 4.2 *Subvalvar pulmonary stenosis*

Subvalvar pulmonary stenosis is rarely isolated, and is more commonly associated with a ventricular septal defect or as part of tetralogy of Fallot. The murmur is related to subvalvar muscle hypertrophy and/or fibrous tissue.

History

History will depend on the severity of the obstruction and the presence of associated cardiac abnormalities. The lesion is usually detected by the presence of a murmur. Severe obstruction may cause shortness of breath on exertion and chest pain.

Examination

There will be no abnormal cardiac physical signs in isolated mild subvalvar pulmonary stenosis other than the murmur. In important subvalvar stenosis there may be a palpable right ventricular impulse and thrill and even signs of right heart failure. Cyanosis may be a feature if there is a large VSD (e.g. in the tetralogy of Fallot) or an ASD.

Heart sounds	S_1, normal
	S_2, soft, normal or loud
Added sounds	Nil
Murmurs	Systolic murmur
Radiation	Pulmonary area and back

ECG
This may be normal, or show right ventricular hypertrophy and possibly right ventricular strain.

CXR
In mild subvalvar pulmonary stenosis the CXR may be normal. In more severe cases there may be cardiomegaly with a right ventricular contour and reduced pulmonary vascularity. In tetralogy of Fallot there may be a right aortic arch and inconspicuous main pulmonary artery.

Echocardiogram
This will define the level of narrowing, and associated abnormalities, such as tetralogy of Fallot. An assessment of the potential for the muscular narrowing to increase in severity can also be made.

Notes

The second heart sound will be quiet in more severe cases. Because the stenosis is usually muscular, the obstruction and the pitch of the murmur increase during systole. In severe cases there may be complete obstruction in the latter part of systole and the murmur will become shorter and softer. In tetralogy of Fallot the aorta is anteriorly placed, so the aortic component of S_2 may be increased. The aortic root is enlarged, so there may also be an aortic ejection click. A pulmonary ejection click is present if there is associated valvar pulmonary stenosis. This murmur is commonly mistaken for a VSD but the murmur of subpulmonary stenosis often radiates to the pulmonary area and through to the back.

Learning point

- The murmur of subpulmonary stenosis may be similar to a VSD
- In tetralogy of Fallot the murmur arises from the subpulmonary stenosis and not the VSD

Summary

• Where is the murmur loudest?	→	Mid left sternal edge
• When does the murmur occur?	→	Systole
• What else could it be?	→	Ventricular septal defect
• What makes it subvalvar pulmonary stenosis?	→	Radiation to the back and rising pitch in systole

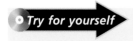

Try for yourself **4.2 Subvalvar pulmonary stenosis**

- Now listen to the recording of subvalvar pulmonary stenosis on the CD. Use these suggestions to ensure that you can hear the murmur. At each step, ensure that you are clear what you are hearing before you move on.

- There is a 2/6 ejection systolic murmur recorded at the mid left sternal edge. Watch the SDC and note that the murmur coincides with it hitting systole. Try to appreciate S_1 and S_2. S_1 is very quiet and S_2 is clear. This murmur could be described as soft, early systolic and occupying three-quarters of systole (hence S_1 is masked by the murmur and S_2 is not). There is no click.

- When you have listened to the native murmur maximize systole to make the murmur louder.

- Watch the SDC and time the heart sounds and the murmur until you are confident that this is a systolic murmur. When you feel confident minimize systole. This will confirm that you were listening to the correct sound, since the systolic murmur has almost disappeared. Now listen to the second heart sound and note that it is clear and widely split. When you feel confident with this, reset and listen again to the native murmur noting the very soft S_1, the clearly audible and split S_2 and the soft systolic murmur.

Quiz

The following statements are true or false. Cover the answers to test your understanding.

1. Subvalvar pulmonary stenosis is usually an isolated condition.
2. The murmur of sub-pulmonary stenosis can be confused with VSD.
3. The murmur of sub-pulmonary stenosis is continuous.
4. Patients with sub-pulmonary stenosis may be cyanosed.
5. Sub-pulmonary stenosis may coexist with valvar pulmonary stenosis.
6. In tetralogy of Fallot, the sub-pulmonary murmur typically becomes louder during a cyanotic spell.
7. The murmur of sub-pulmonary stenosis is loudest in the pulmonary area.
8. In tetralogy of Fallot, the sub-pulmonary murmur typically becomes shorter during a cyanotic spell.
9. Sub-pulmonary stenosis does not usually require treatment.
10. Sub-pulmonary stenosis due to a fibrous ring is less common than that due to muscle.

Answers to quiz

1. False. Subvalvar pulmonary stenosis usually occurs associated with a VSD or as part of tetralogy of Fallot.
2. True. The murmur is in the same place and of similar quality. Sub-pulmonary stenosis more commonly radiates to the back.
3. False. It is systolic and may end before the second heart sound.
4. True. In association with a VSD, for example in tetralogy of Fallot, severe stenosis leads to right to left shunting across the VSD.
5. True. Right ventricular hypertrophy associated with valvar pulmonary stenosis may lead to added subvalvar stenosis.
6. False. Cyanotic spells occur because of increasing dynamic sub-pulmonary stenosis, with decreased flow and a softer or absent murmur.
7. False. Since the murmur arises below the valve, it is loudest at the mid left sternal edge.
8. True. As in 6 above. The increased dynamic sub-pulmonary stenosis allows flow for a shorter time in systole.
9. False. Sub-pulmonary stenosis may be due to muscular hypertrophy, which is dynamic and may lead to life threatening cyanotic 'spells'.
10. True. The occurrence of sub-pulmonary stenosis as part of tetralogy of Fallot makes the muscular form more common.

Pulmonary regurgitation

Anatomy

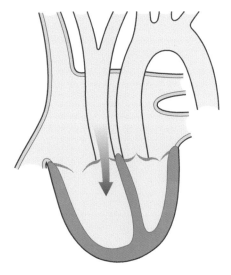

Fig. 4.3 *Pulmonary regurgitation*

Clinically important isolated congenital pulmonary valve regurgitation is rare, although trivial, mild or moderate pulmonary regurgitation is frequently detected by colour flow Doppler imaging during echocardiography. This is not associated with a murmur. Important pulmonary regurgitation is more common after surgery for pulmonary stenosis, particularly in the setting of tetralogy of Fallot.

History

As noted above, there may be a history of surgical or cardiac catheter treatment of a stenotic pulmonary valve. In isolated congenital pulmonary regurgitation, the patient is often symptomatic well into adult life, although the elevation of pulmonary artery pressure due to left ventricular failure, or lung disease may worsen regurgitation through a congenitally abnormal valve. Severe pulmonary hypertension may cause pulmonary regurgitation, even in the presence of a normal valve.

Examination

In mild pulmonary regurgitation the examination will be normal apart from the presence of a murmur. In important pulmonary regurgitation there will be a right ventricular impulse. Right ventricular failure is rare but may occur with chronic severe regurgitation and lead to elevation in the central venous pressure, hepatomegaly and oedema.

Heart sounds	S_1, normal S_2, often widely split
Added sounds	Nil, or pulmonary ejection click
Murmurs	Medium to low-pitched diastolic crescendo-decrescendo murmur

ECG

The ECG is usually normal in pulmonary regurgitation, in the absence of pulmonary hypertension (see Fig. 4.4). There may be signs of right ventricular volume overload. Following surgery for tetralogy of Fallot there will often be complete right bundle branch block.

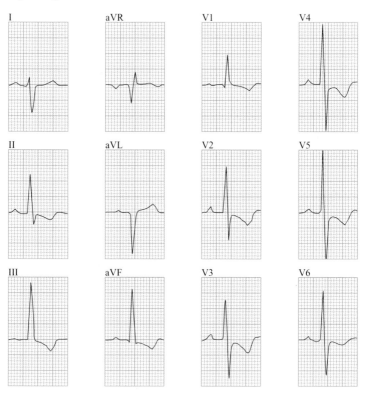

Fig. 4.4 *This patient has severe pulmonary hypertension. There is sinus rhythm with a PR interval at the upper limit of normal (200 ms). There is right axis deviation, common in right ventricular hypertrophy (QRS axis 120 degrees). There are voltage criteria for right ventricular hypertrophy with an almost pure R wave in V1 and a deep S wave in V6. There is also evidence of RV 'strain' with downward-sloping ST depression across the right ventricular leads (in this case extending laterally, across the chest leads, because the right ventricle is hugely dilated)*

CXR

This may be normal in pulmonary regurgitation, in the absence of pulmonary hypertension, or there may be dilatation of the pulmonary trunk (Fig. 4.5). With severe regurgitation there will be enlargement of the right ventricle.

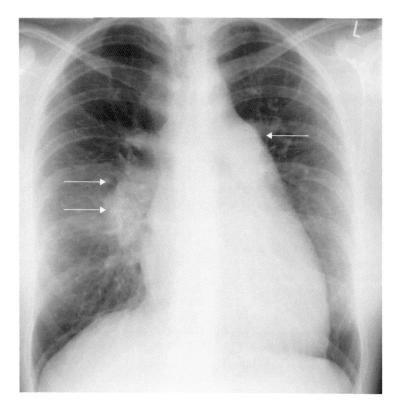

Fig. 4.5 *Pulmonary hypertension. There is cardiomegaly related to a hypertrophied and dilated right ventricle. The pulmonary artery trunk is enlarged (single arrow) as are the proximal branch pulmonary arteries, best seen here on the right (double arrows). Beyond these dilated proximal branch pulmonary arteries there is distal 'pruning', characteristic of pulmonary hypertension*

Echocardiogram

The presence of pulmonary regurgitation is well shown on echocardiogram, but because of the shape of the right ventricle accurate assessment of the severity may be difficult on 2-dimensional echocardiography. This is better done by cardiac MRI or 3D echocardiography.

Notes

The second heart sound is usually widely split due to delay in the pulmonary component, often with right bundle branch block; however, the second heart sound may be single in complete absence of the pulmonary valve. The second heart sound may be closely split if rapid right ventricular ejection is accompanied by a rapid fall in pulmonary artery pressure. The murmur increases in intensity during inspiration.

The murmur is typically mid-diastolic and short in duration. However, in pulmonary hypertension there is a large pressure difference throughout diastole and the murmur is high pitched, and long, sometimes lasting throughout diastole (Graham Steell murmur).

Learning points

- Pulmonary hypertension may cause pulmonary regurgitation in the presence of a normal pulmonary valve
- Pulmonary regurgitation is common after repair of tetralogy of Fallot

---

Summary

• Where is the murmur loudest?	→	Mid left sternal edge
• When does the murmur occur?	→	Diastole
• What else could it be?	→	Aortic regurgitation, although in the absence of pulmonary hypertension, pulmonary regurgitation is usually lower pitched
• What makes it pulmonary regurgitation?	→	Diastolic timing and quality

4.3 Pulmonary regurgitation

- Now listen to the recording of pulmonary regurgitation on the CD. Use these suggestions to ensure that you can hear the murmur. At each step, ensure that you are clear what you are hearing before you move on.

- This is a recording of pulmonary regurgitation taken at the mid left sternal edge in a patient with moderate pulmonary regurgitation and a normal pulmonary artery pressure.

- There is a soft systolic and diastolic murmur. It is vital to be able to hear the two components of the murmur separately. Most trainees initially perceive the systolic murmur but cannot hear the diastolic component. Now eliminate the diastolic component to hear the difference by minimizing diastole.

- There is now a soft S_1, a soft ejection systolic murmur and a louder S_2. Listen to this for a few cycles and note that there is a clear gap after S_2 where there is silence (i.e. diastole) because the diastolic murmur has been removed. When you feel confident, maximize diastole and focus on the two heart sounds and try to appreciate the murmur after S_2 (when the cursor hits diastole). This is the diastolic component, which is short and early. Repeat these last two steps minimizing and maximizing diastole until you are confident that you can hear the short, early diastolic murmur.

- If you are having problems hearing this, try maximizing diastole and minimizing systole.

- The systolic murmur has almost disappeared and the diastolic murmur is accentuated. Watch the SDC and time the murmur: it is clear that the louder murmur is diastolic. When you are confident listen finally to the native murmur. You should now be able to appreciate both parts of the murmur.

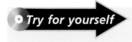 **Try for yourself** **4.4 Pulmonary regurgitation with pulmonary hypertension**

- Now listen to the recording of pulmonary regurgitation with pulmonary hypertension on the CD. This murmur is much louder and higher pitched than the previous one with normal pulmonary artery pressure. Use these suggestions to ensure that you can hear the murmur. At each step, ensure that you are clear what you are hearing before you move on.

- This was also recorded at the mid left sternal edge. In the presence of pulmonary hypertension the higher pitch of the diastolic murmur may make it impossible to differentiate from the murmur of aortic regurgitation. First listen to the native recording. As with all diastolic murmurs, the timing can at first be difficult, so minimize diastole to help appreciate it.

- Watch the SDC. Note that there is now silence in diastole, with S₂ marking the beginning of the silence. When you have listened and feel confident, maximize diastole.

- The diastolic murmur is now really quite loud and dominates the sounds. Listen carefully while watching the SDC. If you are not sure, repeat the last two steps minimizing and maximizing diastole until you feel confident. Finally listen again to the native murmur.

Quiz

The following statements are true or false. Cover the answers to test your understanding.

1. Isolated pulmonary regurgitation is a common congenital abnormality.
2. The predominant murmur in pulmonary regurgitation is systolic.
3. Pulmonary regurgitation may develop in later life due to lung disease.
4. Pulmonary regurgitation seen on echocardiography by colour flow mapping is always important.
5. Mild pulmonary regurgitation is usually symptomatic.
6. A dilated pulmonary artery on chest X-ray may be a sign of PR.
7. In the presence of severe pulmonary hypertension, pulmonary regurgitation may be difficult to distinguish from aortic regurgitation.
8. Pulmonary regurgitation is rare after repair of tetralogy of Fallot.
9. The jugular venous pressure may be elevated in severe PR.
10. The second heart sound may be single in association with PR.

Answers to quiz

1. False. Pulmonary regurgitation is much more common in association with tetralogy of Fallot, or after surgical treatment of pulmonary stenosis.
2. False. Like aortic regurgitation the predominant murmur is diastolic, although a systolic murmur may coexist due to increased RV output, or due to coexistent pulmonary stenosis.
3. True. If bronchopulmonary disease leads to an elevated pulmonary artery pressure, pulmonary regurgitation may develop through a previously normal valve, or associated with pulmonary artery dilatation.
4. False. One study found 42% of 6- to 11-year-olds had trivial to moderate pulmonary regurgitation on colour flow mapping.
5. False. Mild PR is well tolerated and may never become symptomatic.
6. True. A dilated main PA may be the only abnormality on chest X-ray.
7. True. The pitch of the murmur depends on the diastolic pressure in the main pulmonary artery, PR in PHT may be the same pitch as AR.
8. False. Tetralogy of Fallot is associated with an abnormal pulmonary valve, so repair often leads to PR.
9. True. Severe chronic PR will lead to right heart failure and elevation of the jugular venous pressure.
10. True. PR can occur with a very dysplastic, or completely absent pulmonary valve, in which case the second heart sound is singular.

Try for yourself **4.5 Right bundle branch block**

- In right bundle branch block the splitting of the second sound is increased. Although this may occur without an associated ASD, this should always be ruled out.

- Now listen to the recording of right bundle branch block on the CD. Use these suggestions to ensure that you can appreciate the enhanced splitting of the second heart sound. At each step, ensure that you are clear what you are hearing before you move on.

- Listen to the native recording. There is a very soft systolic murmur and there is wide splitting of S_2. Splitting of the second sound, even when it is wide, is a subtle finding. Note that the split S_2 occurs as the SDC hits diastole. In order to concentrate on the second sound, minimize systole.

- You have eliminated the very soft systolic murmur. Try to appreciate the splitting but if you find it difficult, maximize S_2 split.

- Listen carefully and focus on S_2. The systolic murmur is quiet and we have widened the splitting, making it easier to appreciate. When you feel that you have heard the splitting, minimize S_2 split.

- The second sound remains somewhat split, but less so than previously. Repeat the last two steps, maximizing and minimizing the S_2 split until you feel confident.

- Finally listen to the native recording and be sure that you appreciate the splitting of S_2.

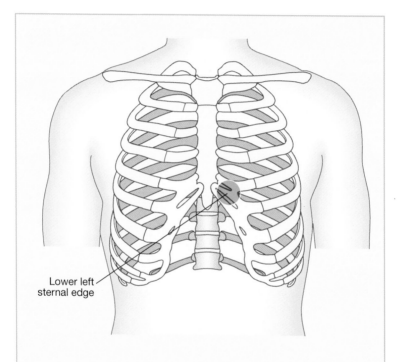

Lower left
sternal edge

The murmurs best heard in this region are:

- Innocent vibratory murmur
- Ventricular septal defect
- Subaortic stenosis
- Tricuspid regurgitation

Innocent vibratory (Still's) murmur

Anatomy

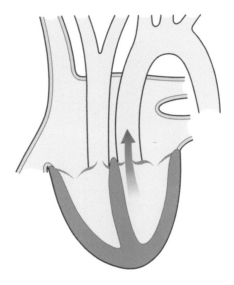

Fig. 5.1 *Innocent vibratory murmur*

This is a very common innocent murmur, most often heard from 3 years of age to adolescence, and by definition the cardiac anatomy is normal. The origin of this murmur is uncertain but it may arise from the left ventricular outflow tract.

History

As the heart is normal there can be no symptoms attributable to the heart. This having been said, the fact that vibratory innocent murmurs are common will mean that in some children with chest pain or breathlessness that is non-cardiac in origin, a murmur may co-exist.

Examination

General and cardiac examination is normal apart from the murmur.

Heart sounds	*Normal*
Added sounds	*Normal*
Murmurs	*Early systolic vibratory murmur*

ECG
The ECG is normal.

CXR
The CXR will be normal.

Echocardiogram
The echocardiogram will confirm a structurally normal heart.

Notes

Innocent vibratory murmurs have a very distinctive sound that has been compared to the twanging of a rubber band. They may be quite loud, up to grade 3/6, but are never associated with a thrill. They occur in early systole and there may be a gap before the second heart sound. They are usually best heard with the patient lying flat and may completely disappear on sitting. They also tend to be more prominent if the patient is febrile or anxious.

Learning points
- Innocent murmurs are very common in childhood
- Classical vibratory murmurs are very distinctive. Occasionally, however, a soft vibratory murmur may be very difficult to differentiate from mild subaortic stenosis

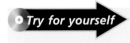

5.1 Vibratory systolic (Still's) murmur

- Now listen to the recording of an innocent vibratory murmur on the CD. Use these suggestions to ensure that you can hear the murmur. At each step, ensure that you are clear what you are hearing before you move on.

- This is a recording taken at the lower left sternal edge. The murmur is early systolic and quite soft. It coincides with the SDC hitting systole. Try to appreciate S_1 and S_2, which are clearly and discretely audible. The main diagnostic feature of this murmur is its quality. Now manipulate the heart sounds to make the murmur easier to hear by maximizing systole.

- If you could not hear the murmur before, it should be more apparent now. S_1 is also now softer than S_2. Watch the SDC and time the two heart sounds. Once you feel confident that you can hear the murmur, minimize systole. Repeat these two steps several times until you feel confident that you have identified the murmur. Finally listen to the native murmur.

Summary		
● Where is the murmur loudest?	→	Lower left sternal edge
● When does the murmur occur?	→	Systole
● What else could it be?	→	Ventricular septal defect or subaortic stenosis
● What makes it a Still's murmur?	→	Position of the murmur, absence of thrill, and quality of the murmur

Quiz

The following statements about innocent vibratory murmurs are true or false. Answer each one and then check the answers below to see if you are correct.

1. Innocent vibratory murmurs are rare in childhood.
2. Innocent murmurs are often louder if a child is febrile.
3. The origin of innocent murmurs is clear on echocardiography.
4. If a child with a murmur has breathlessness, the murmur cannot be innocent.
5. Innocent murmurs are not associated with thrills.
6. Innocent vibratory murmurs have a diastolic component.
7. Innocent vibratory murmurs are best heard at the back.
8. Sub-pulmonary stenosis is a differential diagnosis of an innocent vibratory murmur.
9. Innocent vibratory murmurs radiate to the back.
10. Innocent vibratory murmurs tend to disappear with time.

Answers to quiz

1. False. The peak incidence of innocent murmurs is from 3 years to adolescence.
2. True. They also vary with position and if the patient is anxious.
3. False. There are several theories about the origins of innocent murmurs but none has been proven.
4. False. Although the presence of symptoms which could be cardiac must provoke a careful search to exclude heart disease, the prevalence of innocent murmurs means that they may co-exist with a non-cardiac cause of breathlessness.
5. True. Although innocent vibratory murmurs may be 3/6 in intensity, the presence of a thrill indicates a pathological murmur.
6. False. Innocent vibratory murmurs occur in early systole.
7. False. They are best heard at the lower left sternal edge.
8. False. Sub-aortic stenosis produces a murmur at the lower left sternal edge, and on occasions this may be vibratory in quality.
9. False. Innocent vibratory murmurs may be quite widespread on the precordium, although loudest at the lower left sternal edge, but they do not radiate to the back.
10. True. They are rare after puberty.

Ventricular septal defect

Anatomy

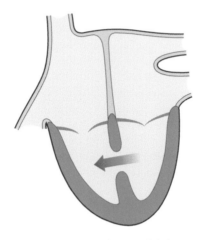

Fig. 5.2 Ventricular septal defect

A ventricular septal defect (VSD) is a hole in the septum between the two ventricles. VSDs may vary in size from pinhole to almost complete absence of the septum, and the physical signs vary accordingly. The position of the defect is perimembranous (around the membranous septum adjacent to the aortic and tricuspid valves) or muscular (anywhere else). Perimembranous defects may extend into part of the muscular septum, and while the position cannot usually be distinguished clinically, sub-arterial defects may sometimes be appreciated (see later) (Fig. 5.3). Ventricular septal defects may be single or multiple, and when multiple, they may be muscular, or a perimembranous defect may coexist with single or multiple muscular defects. Ventricular septal defects may also occur as part of more complex congenital heart disease, and in this case they may not give rise to murmurs because of equal left and right ventricular pressures. We will therefore be considering the murmur associated with an isolated VSD.

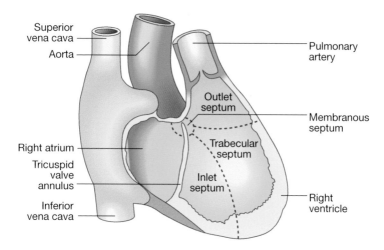

Fig. 5.3 *Ventricular septum shown from right ventricular side (modified from* Clinical Recognition of Congenital Heart Disease, *5th edition, by Joseph K Perloff, 2003, Saunders)*

History

The presentation of a VSD or VSDs will depend upon their overall size, the shunt associated with them and the pulmonary vascular resistance. Small defects are diagnosed because of a murmur heard on routine examination soon after birth. Small defects, particularly in the muscular septum have a tendency to undergo spontaneous closure, so such murmurs may disappear. Moderate or large defects may not result in a murmur immediately after birth because of a delay in the normal fall in the pulmonary vascular resistance. They will then present with 'heart failure' in the first few months of life. This manifests as breathlessness, sweatiness and failure to gain weight in infancy. These symptoms may lead to surgical or medical treatment. With time the overall left-to-right shunt will decrease, either due to reduction in size of the defect or to increased pulmonary vascular resistance (PVR). If untreated, a continuing rise in pulmonary vascular resistance will eventually lead to a suprasystemic PVR, with shunt reversal and cyanosis (Eisenmenger's syndrome).

Examination

General examination should as always include an assessment for dysmorphic features because VSDs are associated with many syndromes (e.g. trisomy 21, trisomy 13, Holt Oram syndrome and fetal alcohol syndrome). There may be no abnormal cardiac physical signs in a small VSD other than a cardiac murmur, although a thrill is not uncommon. This is best felt at the left sternal border in the third or fourth intercostal space, unless the defect is subarterial, in which case it is felt at the first or second intercostal space. In moderate defects there will be signs of left ventricular volume overload, including a prominent left ventricular impulse which may be displaced, and a mitral diastolic flow murmur. Large defects may present with heart failure early in life, so the infant may be underweight and frail with obvious breathlessness at rest. An older child may show Harrison's sulci due to chronic dyspnoea and the jugular venous pulse may be elevated. If there is pulmonary hypertension, the patient may be cyanosed and clubbed, with the VSD signs replaced by those of pulmonary hypertension.

Small ventricular septal defect

Heart sounds	S_1, normal
	S_2, normal
Added sounds	Nil
Murmurs	Pansystolic murmur, or early systolic murmur if smaller

Moderate ventricular septal defect

Heart sounds	S_1, normal
	S_2, normal or accentuated
Added sounds	Nil, or third heart sound
Murmurs	Systole: pansystolic murmur
	Diastole: mitral flow murmur

Ventricular septal defect with Eisenmenger syndrome

Heart sounds	S_1, normal
	S_2, loud and single
Added sounds	Nil, or third heart sound
Murmurs	Systole: VSD murmur disappears when shunt reverses
	Diastole: may be pulmonary regurgitation murmur

ECG

The ECG will be normal in small defects, but will demonstrate voltage criteria for left ventricular or biventricular hypertrophy in medium to large defects. Broad notched p waves may be present with large shunts. With the onset of pulmonary hypertension, right ventricular hypertrophy will predominate. These findings are independent of the site of the defect and merely reflect the size of the shunt and the right ventricular pressure. The presence of a septal aneurysm in association with a perimembranous defect may lead to conduction abnormalities and rhythm disturbances.

CXR

This will be normal in small defects. Moderate defects will cause left atrial and left ventricular dilatation with pulmonary plethora. The pulmonary artery may also be prominent. With the onset of pulmonary hypertension, peripheral pruning of pulmonary vessels may become evident with an enlarged right ventricle.

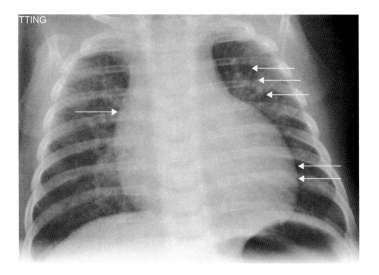

Fig. 5.4 *This infant has a ventricular septal defect. There is a prominent thymic shadow (arrow). The heart is enlarged and the left contour is rounded suggesting a dilated left ventricle (double arrows). The pulmonary vascular markings are prominent indicating a left-to-right shunt (triple arrows)*

Echocardiogram

The echocardiogram will define the position of the defect in the ventricular septum. An assessment of size, overall shunt and pulmonary artery pressure can be made and these will inform the need for treatment. The presence of other abnormalities, such as obstruction to the left or right heart will also be assessed.

Notes

As a VSD becomes smaller the murmur becomes shorter because the defect closes before the end of systole. The murmur may also be highly localized on the chest wall. In moderate VSDs with large left to right shunts there may be mid-systolic accentuation of the murmur due to a pulmonary flow component, and similarly there may be a mitral diastolic flow murmur. Perimembranous VSDs may be associated with aortic regurgitation. Subaortic stenosis may cause a similar murmur to a small VSD but radiates to the aortic area. Similarly, subpulmonary stenosis may be confused with a VSD but the murmur radiates to the pulmonary area and through to the back. The murmur of tricuspid regurgitation is similar to that of a small VSD.

Learning points

- Subaortic stenosis may masquerade as a VSD
- Perimembranous VSDs may be associated with aortic regurgitation
- Small VSDs may cause a loud murmur
- Large VSDs may only cause a soft murmur

Summary

• Where is the murmur loudest?	→	Lower left sternal edge
• When does the murmur occur?	→	Systole
• What else could it be?	→	Subvalvar pulmonary or aortic stenosis, innocent Still's murmur
• What makes it a VSD?	→	Quality of the murmur

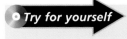

Try for yourself 5.2 Loud muscular ventricular septal defect

- Now listen to the recording of a loud muscular ventricular septal defect on the CD. Use these suggestions to help you to hear the murmur. At each step, ensure that you are clear what you are hearing before you move on.

- The murmur of a large muscular VSD may be described as a blowing systolic murmur and this one is of 3/6 intensity and occupies three-quarters of systole. Watch the SDC and note that the murmur coincides with it hitting systole. Try to appreciate S_2, which is clearly audible (i.e. the murmur does not run into S_2 and therefore the murmur is not pansystolic). Now manipulate the heart sounds to ensure that you are listening to the murmur. First minimize systole. This greatly diminishes the systolic murmur but does not completely eliminate it. This allows you to focus on the heart sounds. S_1 is slightly softer than S_2. Watch the SDC and time the two heart sounds. When you feel that you have identified S_1 and S_2, maximize S_2. This will confirm that you have identified the sounds correctly.

- Next minimize S_2 and maximize systole. Listen to the systolic murmur and note that S_2 is now inaudible. Because S_2 is now inaudible the murmur sounds pansystolic. (Murmurs in VSDs are often described in textbooks as pansystolic, but this is not always the case.)

- Finally listen to the native murmur and again confirm that the murmur does not in fact reach S_2, which is clearly audible. Remember—not all VSD murmurs are pansystolic!

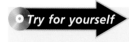 **Try for yourself** **5.3 Very small muscular ventricular septal defect**

- Now listen to the recording of a very small muscular ventricular septal defect on the CD. Use these suggestions to help you to hear the murmur. At each step, ensure that you are clear what you are hearing before you move on.

- This is a blowing systolic murmur of 2/6 intensity which occupies three-quarters of systole. Watch the SDC and note that the murmur coincides with it hitting systole. Try to appreciate S_2, which is clearly audible as in the previous example. Now manipulate the heart sounds to appreciate the murmur more easily. First minimize systole to eliminate the systolic murmur and allow you to focus on the heart sounds. S_1 is slightly softer than S_2. Watch the SDC and time the two heart sounds.

- Once you feel that you have identified S_1 and S_2, confirm this by maximizing S_2, then minimize S_2 and maximize systole.

- As in the previous example, this simulates a pansystolic murmur as in the classical description of a VSD murmur. After listening to this reset to the native murmur and confirm that S_2 is audible and the murmur is not in fact pansystolic.

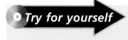 **Try for yourself** **5.4 Perimembranous ventricular septal defect**

- Now listen to the recording of a perimembranous ventricular septal defect on the CD. Use these suggestions to help you to hear the murmur. At each step, ensure that you are clear what you are hearing before you move on.

- This is a blowing systolic murmur of 3/6 intensity which occupies three-quarters of systole. Watch the SDC and note that the murmur coincides with it hitting systole. In this example, as in the previous two, S_2 is clearly audible and the murmur is not pansystolic. Now manipulate the heart sounds to ensure that you have identified the two heart sounds and the murmur. First minimize systole. By eliminating the systolic murmur you can focus on the heart sounds. S_1 is slightly softer than S_2. Watch the SDC and time the two heart sounds. When you feel confident that you have identified the two heart sounds correctly, check by maximizing S_2. Following this, simulate a pansystolic murmur as in the two previous examples by minimizing S_2 and maximizing systole.

- When you have appreciated what a pansystolic murmur would sound like, listen to the native murmur and again confirm that the murmur does not in fact reach S_2, which is clearly audible.

Quiz

The following statements about ventricular septal defects are true or false. Answer each one and then check the answers below to see if you are correct.

1. The typical murmur of a VSD is systolic.
2. Large VSDs may be associated with diastolic murmurs.
3. All VSD murmurs sound the same.
4. The larger the VSD, the louder the murmur.
5. Muscular VSDs always require surgical closure.
6. Muscular VSD murmurs may be soft and very localized.
7. All VSDs requiring closure will have typical systolic murmurs.
8. VSD murmurs are more common in babies than in older children.
9. The murmur heard in tetralogy of Fallot is due to the VSD.
10. VSD murmurs are typically heard at the apex.

Answers to quiz

1. True. The typical murmur of a VSD is a long systolic murmur, although not always pansystolic.
2. True. Large VSDs are associated with mitral flow murmurs.
3. False. Muscular VSDs may close before the end of systole leading to a rise in pitch at the end of the murmur. This does not happen with perimembranous VSDs.
4. False. Very large VSDs may not be associated with murmurs, and in the setting of pulmonary hypertension the murmur may be soft or absent.
5. False. VSDs in general have a tendency to get smaller with time and some undergo complete spontaneous closure.
6. True. Small muscular VSDs may have very soft murmurs in a very precise location relating to the position of the VSD in the septum.
7. False. Particularly in young babies, a large VSD may be associated with a delay in fall of the pulmonary vascular resistance and little or no systolic murmur.
8. True. This is because VSDs, particularly muscular ones, tend to undergo spontaneous closure.
9. False. Because the VSD is unrestrictive, and the ventricular pressures are equal, there is no VSD murmur in tetralogy. The murmur is due to sub-pulmonary and pulmonary stenosis.
10. False. A systolic murmur heard at the apex is due to mitral regurgitation.

Subaortic stenosis

Anatomy

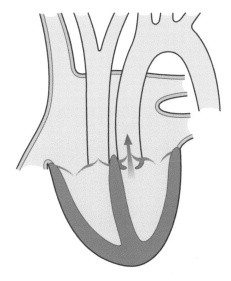

Fig. 5.5 *Subaortic stenosis*

Subaortic stenosis is most commonly caused by a fibrous crescent-shaped membrane, although a longer fibromuscular tunnel is not uncommon. It may be isolated, or associated with other congenital abnormalities, particularly an abnormal aortic or mitral valve, and in association with a VSD. Sub-aortic obstruction may also be dynamic, due to muscular thickening in the setting of hypertrophic obstructive cardiomyopathy (HOCM).

History

Subaortic stenosis due to a fibromuscular membrane is rare in infancy, and commonest in childhood and young adulthood. In older patients it is more likely to be muscular in the setting of HOCM. The patient may be asymptomatic despite severe obstruction, although tiredness on exercise and syncope on exercise are worrying symptoms. Angina is not uncommon in important obstruction.

Examination

In mild obstruction the examination will be normal apart from the presence of a murmur. The arterial pulse may be of small volume in important subaortic obstruction. There may also be a thrill in the suprasternal notch and over the carotid arteries, and this may be present at the mid left sternal edge (mimicking that of a VSD). In severe obstruction there may be a left ventricular heave. Aortic regurgitation can develop with subaortic obstruction so this murmur may also be audible.

Heart sounds	S_1, normal
	S_2, normal or soft
Added sounds	Usually nil. There may be a fourth heart sound
Murmurs	Long systolic murmur which radiates to the aortic area

ECG

The ECG is normal in mild obstruction. Left ventricular forces are increased in important obstruction and there may be repolarization changes. If HOCM is the underlying cause, then the ECG feature of this will predominate.

CXR

This may be normal even with severe obstruction. The ascending aorta is not dilated, in contrast to valvar aortic stenosis.

Echocardiogram

The nature of the obstruction will be defined, together with the severity of obstruction, judged by the gradient across the left ventricular outflow tract, and the presence of any associated aortic regurgitation.

Notes

The aortic component of the second sound becomes quieter as the degree of obstruction increases. The murmur is different in quality to that of valvar aortic stenosis, the thrill and area of maximum intensity of the murmur are at the lower left sternal edge and there is no valvar click, so the murmur is more likely to be mistaken for a VSD than for valvar aortic stenosis.

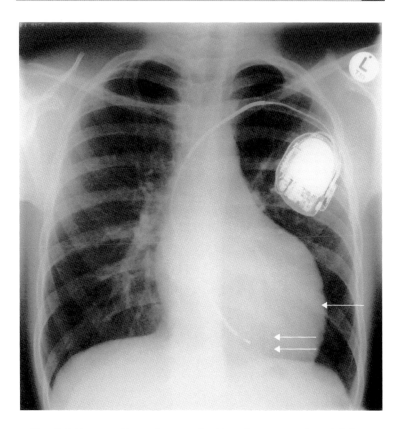

Fig. 5.6 Hypertrophic cardiomyopathy. Note the very prominent left heart border indicating severe left ventricular hypertrophy (single arrow). This patient has an implantable defibrillator because of a previous out-of-hospital cardiac arrest. The lead has been placed through the innominate vein and into the right ventricular apex (double arrows)

Learning points

- Aortic regurgitation is present in about 50% of cases
- Subaortic obstruction may be progressive
- Subaortic obstruction may be confused with a VSD

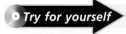 **Try for yourself** **5.5 Subvalvar aortic stenosis**

- Now listen to the recording of subvalvar aortic stenosis on the CD. Use these suggestions to help you to hear the murmur. At each step, ensure that you are clear what you are hearing before you move on.

- This murmur was recorded at the lower left sternal edge. It is blowing and long but does not reach S_2, which is clearly heard. When you have listened to the native murmur, and identified S_1 and S_2, minimize S_2. This allows you to be sure that you had identified S_2. It also simulates a pansystolic murmur. Note the similarity to a VSD murmur.

- When you have appreciated this maximize S_2 and hear that it is audible after the end of the murmur.

- Next minimize systole to almost abolish the murmur and make the heart sounds clearly audible. Finally listen again to the native murmur.

Summary		
● Where is the murmur loudest?	→	Lower left sternal edge
● When does the murmur occur?	→	Systole
● What else could it be?	→	Innocent murmur, VSD, tricuspid regurgitation
● What makes it subaortic stenosis?	→	Radiation to aortic area

Quiz

The following statements are true or false. Cover the answers to test your understanding.

1. The murmur of subaortic stenosis may be mistaken for a VSD.
2. There may be a diastolic murmur associated with a sub AS murmur.
3. The murmur of sub AS is best heard at the upper left sternal edge.
4. The murmur of subaortic stenosis may become louder with time.
5. A systolic murmur at the lower left sternal edge after surgical removal of a subaortic membrane can safely be ignored.
6. Development of a diastolic murmur in a patient known to have a subaortic membrane may be due to bacterial endocarditis.
7. Subaortic obstruction may cause angina.
8. The pulse is typically wide volume in isolated subaortic obstruction.
9. Subaortic obstruction may occur with HOCM.
10. Subaortic obstruction may occur in complex congenital heart disease.

Answers to quiz

1. True. The murmur is loudest at the lower left sternal edge and may have a similar quality to a VSD.
2. True. Aortic regurgitation is present echocardiographically in 50% of cases of subaortic stenosis.
3. False. Although the murmur of aortic stenosis is best heard at the upper left sternal edge, that of subaortic stenosis is loudest lower on the chest.
4. True. Subaortic stenosis may progress and the murmur will become louder until severe obstruction leads to reduced cardiac output.
5. False. Subaortic membranes may recur and therefore continued follow-up is necessary, and recurrent murmurs should be investigated.
6. True. Although aortic regurgitation may develop and progress in the absence of endocarditis, subaortic obstruction does predispose to bacterial endocarditis, so a new murmur should raise this possibility.
7. True. This may be due to left ventricular hypertrophy and limited cardiac output to the coronary arteries from the obstruction.
8. False. Typically the pulse is small volume with isolated obstruction.
9. True. There may also be mitral regurgitation.
10. True. It is associated with coarctation and mitral stenosis, double outlet right ventricle or complex single ventricle circulation.

Tricuspid regurgitation

Anatomy

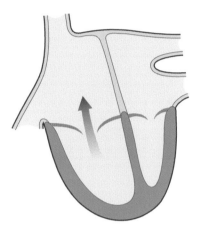

Fig. 5.7 Tricuspid regurgitation

Isolated tricuspid regurgitation is most common with Ebstein's anomaly of the tricuspid valve, in which the septal leaflet of the valve is attached further down the ventricular septum than normal. The degree of tricuspid regurgitation ranges from mild to torrential. Tricuspid regurgitation may also result from a congenitally dysplastic valve and occasionally after spontaneous closure of a VSD when the septal leaflet of the tricuspid valve becomes adherent to the margins of the defect. Tricuspid regurgitation may also occur if an anatomically normal valve becomes stretched as a result of right heart dilatation, for example, due to an atrial septal defect or after surgery for tetralogy of Fallot.

History

Severe tricuspid regurgitation may lead to fetal hydrops or even death in utero. The patient may present in early infancy with cyanosis, breathlessness and low cardiac output. In less severe cases the diagnosis may be made because of the murmur, the presence of cyanosis, which may deepen with time, or palpitations or syncope due to atrial arrhythmias. The presence of a right to left shunt through the atrial communication leads to the risk of paradoxical embolism. Patients may, however, be asymptomatic well into adult life.

Examination

There may be central cyanosis. This is related to the atrial communication which is present in the majority of patients with Ebstein's anomaly. Cyanosis is common immediately after birth, and may resolve as the pulmonary vascular resistance falls. It may recur later in life when right ventricular filling pressure rises. Some patients have ruddy cheeks. The jugular venous pulse is normal until right ventricular failure occurs. This is due to the compliant right atrium and atrialized portion of the right ventricle. In Ebstein's anomaly there may be no right ventricular heave, but this is usually present when tricuspid regurgitation is due to other causes. Similarly, a pulsatile liver is rare in Ebstein's anomaly, but more common in severe tricuspid regurgitation from other causes.

Heart sounds	S_1, normal or loud. May be widely split in Ebstein's anomaly or may appear single due to a quiet mitral component S_2, normal, single or may be widely split
Added sounds	Nil, S_3 and S_4 may be heard
Murmurs	Early systolic/pansystolic murmur

ECG

The PR interval may be short, normal or prolonged. Pre-excitation is present in 25% of patients with Ebstein's anomaly and the P wave is usually tall. The QRS complex is usually prolonged and shows a right bundle branch block pattern.

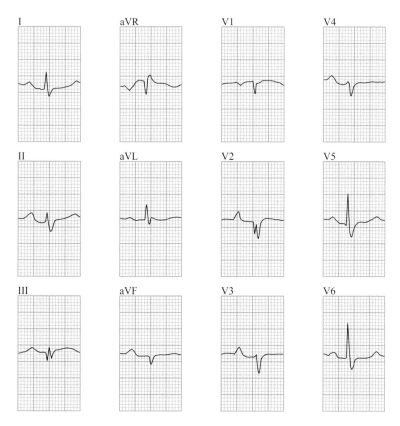

Fig. 5.8 *This patient has Ebstein's anomaly of the tricuspid valve with severe tricuspid regurgitation. The main feature is right atrial hypertrophy: this is characterized by a prolonged P wave duration (120 ms), and increased P wave voltages particularly notable in this ECG in leads II, V2 and V3. Classically, the best lead to assess for right atrial hypertrophy is lead II*

CXR

The cardiac contour may be normal or enlarged, sometimes massively so. The pulmonary vascularity is either normal or decreased. The pulmonary trunk is inconspicuous in Ebstein's anomaly, but will be enlarged if the tricuspid regurgitation is the result of an ASD or is associated with pulmonary regurgitation.

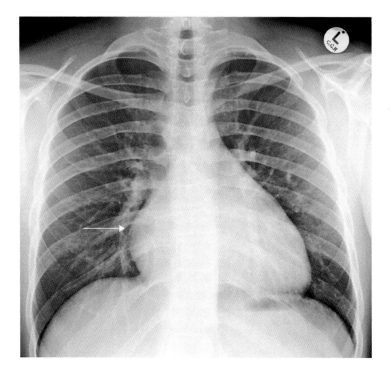

Fig. 5.9 *Ebstein's anomaly of the tricuspid valve. Note the cardiomegaly, usually due to a massively dilated right atrium (arrow, secondary to severe tricuspid regurgitation). The pulmonary artery trunk is small and there is a degree of oligaemia*

Echocardiogram

The anatomy of the tricuspid valve, and so the mechanism of regurgitation, will be demonstrated. As with pulmonary regurgitation (Chapter 4) the severity of regurgitation may be better assessed using cardiac MRI or 3D echocardiography.

Notes

The murmur can vary in length from early systolic to pansystolic. In Ebstein's anomaly the first heart sound is widely split due to the delay in closure of the large anterior leaflet, although this may not be appreciated due to the soft mitral component of the first heart sound. The second sound may similarly appear single due to a soft pulmonary component caused by a low pressure in the pulmonary trunk. The presence of pre-excitation on the ECG in Ebstein's may lead to para-doxical splitting of the second heart sound. The murmur of tricuspid regurgitation varies with respiration if the right ventricle is functioning well. However, in Ebstein's anomaly the poorly functioning small right ventricle cannot usually accommodate the increased venous return on inspiration so the murmur does not alter.

Summary

● Where is the murmur loudest?	→	Lower left sternal edge
● When does the murmur occur?	→	Systole
● What else could it be?	→	VSD or subaortic stenosis
● What makes it tricuspid regurgitation?	→	Quality and variation with respiration

●Try for yourself   5.6 Tricuspid regurgitation

- Listen to the recording of tricuspid regurgitation. Use these suggestions to help you to hear the murmur. At each step, ensure that you are clear what you are hearing before you move on.

- This recording was made at the lower left sternal edge. First listen to the native recording and try to identify the murmur. Next maximize systole to make the murmur more obvious. After listening for a few cardiac cycles, minimize systole to almost abolish the murmur. It can be easier to appreciate the murmur after listening without it present. Repeat these two steps until you are confident that you can hear the tricuspid regurgitation murmur. Finally listen to the native recording.

Quiz

The following statements are true or false. Cover the answers to test your understanding.

1. Tricuspid regurgitation may occur after spontaneous closure of a VSD.
2. Ebstein's anomaly is universally fatal in childhood.
3. The murmur of TR classically is enhanced by inspiration.
4. Tricuspid regurgitation is typically quieter than mitral regurgitation.
5. Tricuspid regurgitation is a diastolic murmur.
6. There may be pre-excitation visible on the ECG is Ebstein's anomaly.
7. Atrial communications are rare in association with Ebstein's anomaly.
8. Tricuspid regurgitation may occur after surgery for tetralogy of Fallot.
9. The heart may be very enlarged on the CXR with tricuspid regurgitation.
10. The liver may be enlarged and pulsatile with severe TR.

Answers to quiz

1. True. The septal leaflet of the tricuspid valve may become adherent to the site of the VSD leading to regurgitation.
2. False. Although Ebstein's anomaly may be fatal in infancy, presentation is variable and some people are asymptomatic into adulthood.
3. True. Although as noted, this may not occur is some cases of Ebstein's anomaly, or if there is right ventricular failure.
4. True. This is because the right ventricle is typically a low pressure chamber. This will not be the case if there is pulmonary hypertension.
5. False. Tricuspid regurgitation is systolic.
6. True. There may be multiple accessory pathways in Ebstein's anomaly. Supraventricular tachycardia may be the first presentation of Ebstein's anomaly.
7. False. They are common in association with Ebstein's anomaly. This may be because the tricuspid regurgitation stretches the right atrium and does not allow the PFO to close.
8. True. Tricuspid and pulmonary regurgitation occur after repair of tetralogy.
9. True. Particularly in Ebstein's anomaly, when the right atrium and atrialized portion of the right ventricle may be very dilated.
10. True. This is true if right ventricular function is good. In Ebstein's anomaly, pulsatility may be lost due to poor right ventricular function.

Apex

6

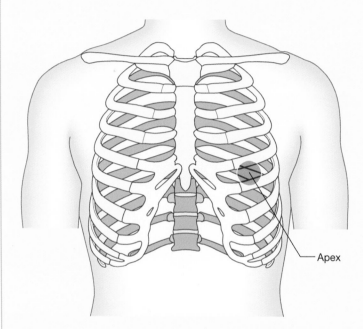

The apex is between the mid-clavicular line and the anterior axillary line in the fifth intercostal space on the left

The murmurs best heard in this region are:
- Mitral regurgitation
- Mitral valve prolapse
- Mitral valve stenosis

Mitral regurgitation

Anatomy

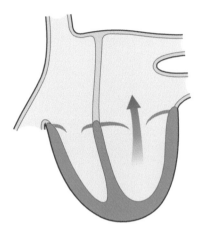

Fig. 6.1 *Mitral regurgitation*

Isolated mitral regurgitation is rare in childhood, and in paediatric practice it is usually associated with atrioventricular septal defects. In adulthood it is more common and often associated with ischaemic heart disease in the setting of reduced left ventricular function, when it is often referred to as 'functional' mitral regurgitation resulting from mitral annular dilatation. Other causes include rheumatic valve disease, degenerative mitral valve disease, mitral valve dysplasia, congenital clefts in the mitral valve leaflets (usually the anterior leaflet) and in association with parachute mitral valve. When mitral regurgitation is present, the left ventricle becomes volume loaded (i.e. there is an increase in pre-load) because the ventricle has to accommodate, in diastole, the normal pulmonary venous return plus the regurgitant volume. The left ventricular end diastolic volume increases and, if unchecked, can lead to myocardial dysfunction. The aim of follow-up is to intervene before this stage is reached.

History

Mild to moderate mitral regurgitation is not usually associated with symptoms but effort intolerance and breathlessness will supervene as it progresses. If there is chordal rupture, there is a sudden onset of breathlessness and fatigue due to acute mitral regurgitation. After myocardial infarction, the papillary muscle may rupture, and this leads to acute severe mitral regurgitation, which is combined with the impaired left ventricular function caused by the myocardial infarction, and has a very poor prognosis.

Examination

On examination, in mild cases, the murmur will be the only abnormal cardiac physical sign. As the degree of mitral regurgitation progresses a prominent apical impulse will be apparent and this will become displaced towards and beyond the anterior axillary line in more severe cases. There is a sinus tachycardia to maintain the cardiac output, unless the cause is rheumatic, in which case there is a high incidence of atrial dysrhythmia. There may be an apical thrill in severe regurgitation. The pulse is 'jerky' due to the fast upstroke. Severe mitral regurgitation is a cause of congestive cardiac failure, which will be manifest by the usual signs and symptoms.

Heart sounds	*Normal*
Added sounds	*None, S_3, S_4, S_3+S_4 (gallop rhythm)*
Murmurs	*Systolic (not 'ejection')*
	Associated diastolic murmur in severe cases

ECG

The ECG is usually normal in mild to moderate mitral regurgitation but, as the severity increases, voltage criteria for left ventricular hypertrophy may develop. Repolarization abnormalities (ST depression and T wave inversion in the infero-lateral leads) may be associated with important mitral regurgitation.

CXR

This will be normal in mild mitral regurgitation. As the degree of mitral regurgitation becomes haemodynamically significant, the left atrium will enlarge and be associated with splaying of the carina. The left ventricular contour will become more prominent (a 'rounding off' of the apex) and cardiomegaly will be apparent. In acute mitral regurgitation there may be pulmonary oedema. The raised left atrial pressure leads to pulmonary venous hypertension which may be recognised on the chest X-ray.

Echocardiogram

The echocardiogram will define the anatomy of the mitral valve and so the mechanism of the mitral regurgitation. An assessment of left ventricular function, and pulmonary artery pressure may be made. The severity of the regurgitation may be assessed using colour flow mapping.

Notes

The murmur of mitral regurgitation is systolic and starts at the onset of systole (compare this to the special case of mitral regurgitation associated with mitral valve prolapse, when the murmur may be late systolic). The intensity relates reasonably well to the severity, but be aware that severe mitral regurgitation can be associated with a quiet murmur, particularly when there is left ventricular dysfunction. The murmur can occupy any proportion of systole but is classically described as a 'pansystolic' or 'holosystolic' murmur. The less severe the mitral regurgitation the shorter the murmur tends to be, so that in very mild cases it will be soft and early systolic. If left ventricular dysfunction supervenes, added sounds will appear and eventually a gallop rhythm may develop. In moderate and severe cases of mitral regurgitation there is increased *diastolic* flow across the mitral valve and, as a result, an apical mitral *diastolic* murmur may be heard which is similar to that associated with mitral stenosis.

Learning points

- The murmur of mitral regurgitation begins with S_1
- The murmur of mitral regurgitation is classically but not necessarily pansystolic
- A soft murmur does not always represent mild disease
- A mitral diastolic murmur (in the absence of mitral stenosis) indicates important regurgitation
- Acute severe mitral regurgitation causes pulmonary oedema and a murmur may be absent

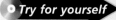 **6.1 Mitral regurgitation**

- Listen to the recording of mitral regurgitation on the CD. Use the following suggestions to ensure that you have identified the murmur correctly. There is a soft systolic murmur representing mild mitral regurgitation which was recorded at the apex. The first heart sound is audible and the murmur begins just after this. The second heart sound marks the end of the murmur. Try to appreciate the murmur before we reduce its intensity.

- Minimize systole so that the heart sounds are clear but the murmur has disappeared. As you listen, watch the SDC to time the heart sounds. When you feel confident, maximize systole and listen again.

- The murmur is now louder and more easily appreciated. Repeat the steps of minimizing and maximizing systole until you are confident of the murmur.

- Finally listen to the native murmur.

Summary

● Where is the murmur loudest?	→	Apex
● When does the murmur occur?	→	Systole
● What else could it be?	→	VSD
● What makes it mitral regurgitation?	→	Position of the apex

Mitral valve prolapse

Anatomy

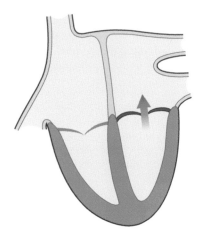

Fig. 6.2 *Mitral valve prolapse*

Mitral valve prolapse is a specific disorder of the mitral valve papillary muscles resulting in a lack of support of one or both leaflets and varying degrees of mitral regurgitation. It is more common in females and the overall incidence is probably around 2 to 3% but depends on the criteria used to define prolapse. It is also more common in connective tissue disorders, such as Ehlers–Danlos syndrome, and Marfan syndrome, when it may be associated with aortic root dilatation.

History

It has been suggested that atypical chest pain is more common in people with mitral valve prolapse. Rare patients with mitral valve prolapse will develop acute chordal rupture. Symptoms will depend on the degree and rate of progression of secondary mitral regurgitation and the notes above will equally apply here. Mitral valve prolapse does increase the risk of bacterial endocarditis.

Examination

There is frequently a systolic click reflecting the movement of the valve cusps into the left atrium in systole, and the murmur of mitral regurgitation immediately follows this. The classical case will therefore have an apical systolic click and late systolic murmur. However, in minor cases there may be a click without a murmur, making it difficult to differentiate it from the ejection click associated with a bicuspid aortic valve, which is also often loudest at the apex. Furthermore, severe mitral valve prolapse may be associated with a pansystolic murmur of mitral regurgitation without a click: echocardiography is necessary to make the diagnosis of mitral valve prolapse in these cases. See notes above on mitral regurgitation.

Heart sounds	*Normal*
Added sounds	*None, systolic click, S_3, S_4, S_3+S_4 (gallop rhythm)*
Murmurs	*None, late systolic or pansystolic*
	Associated diastolic murmur in severe cases

ECG

As for mitral regurgitation.

CXR

As for mitral regurgitation.

Echocardiogram

The diagnosis of mitral valve prolapse is made on echocardiography, and associated mitral regurgitation may be assessed as above.

Learning points

- Mitral valve prolapse is a specific cause of mitral regurgitation
- Mitral valve prolapse is usually associated with an apical systolic click and late systolic murmur
- Mitral valve prolapse can present with acute chordal rupture
- Look for signs of the Marfan syndrome and other connective tissue disorders

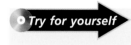 **6.2 Mitral valve prolapse with ejection click and soft systolic murmur**

- Listen to the recording of mitral valve prolapse on the CD. Use the suggestions to ensure that you have correctly identified the mitral valve click followed by the mitral regurgitation murmur. First listen to the native murmur. The click follows S_1 and can be mistaken for a split S_1. There is a soft systolic murmur which begins towards the end of systole, the typical late systolic murmur of mitral valve prolapse. S_2 marks the end of the murmur.

- Next minimize systole. The heart sounds are clear but the click and the murmur have disappeared. As you listen, watch the SDC to time the heart sounds. When you have listened for a few cardiac cycles maximize systole.

- The systolic click has returned and the murmur is now reasonably loud. Try to appreciate the click followed by the murmur. Repeat the last two steps minimizing and maximizing systole until you are confident that you have identified the click and the murmur. Finally listen to the native recording and see that you can still hear the click and the murmur.

Summary		
● Where is the murmur loudest?	→	Apex
● When does the murmur occur?	→	Systole
● What else could it be?	→	The click could be from the aortic valve; the murmur could be a ventricular septal defect
● What makes it mitral valve prolapse?	→	The association of a click and murmur, loudest at the apex

Quiz

The following statements are true or false. Cover the answers to test your understanding.

1. The murmur of mitral regurgitation is always pansystolic.
2. There may be a diastolic murmur with severe mitral regurgitation.
3. Mitral valve prolapse is more common in men.
4. The murmur of MR is loudest at the lower left sternal edge.
5. An apical pansystolic murmur may occur with a partial AVSD.
6. Acute MR is a relatively benign complication of myocardial infarction.
7. Rheumatic fever may lead to mitral regurgitation.
8. Mitral regurgitation is more common in childhood than adulthood.
9. Mitral valve prolapse may be present in more than one member of the same family.
10. The click of mitral valve prolapse may be mistaken for an aortic click.

Answers to quiz

1. False. In severe disease, the LA pressure may equalize with the LV pressure during systole and the murmur stops before the end of systole.
2. True. The extra flow may cause a mitral diastolic flow murmur.
3. False. Mitral valve prolapse is more common in women.
4. False. It is best heard at the apex. A systolic murmur best heard at the lower left sternal edge is likely to be tricuspid regurgitation or a VSD.
5. True. The atrioventricular valves are abnormal in atrioventricular septal defect and so regurgitation is common.
6. False. Acute mitral regurgitation following myocardial infarction is due to papillary muscle rupture and combined with impaired left ventricular function has a poor prognosis.
7. True. The mitral valve may be stenotic, regurgitant, or both following rheumatic fever.
8. False. The incidence of mitral regurgitation rises with age due to 'functional' mitral regurgitation and degenerative mitral valve disease.
9. True. Because mitral valve prolapse is associated with Marfan syndrome it may be present in several members of the same family.
10. True. The click of mitral prolapse is best heard at the apex, as is that of a bicuspid aortic valve.

Mitral valve stenosis

Anatomy

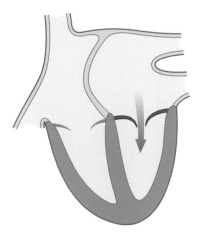

Fig. 6.3 *Mitral valve stenosis*

In adult practice, mitral valve stenosis is usually rheumatic in origin and associated with mitral regurgitation. In childhood, isolated mitral stenosis is extremely rare and results from congenital abnormalities of the mitral valve (e.g. parachute mitral valve), or is due to a supravalvar membrane. Mitral stenosis or atresia as part of hypoplastic left heart syndrome will present as a collapsed neonate and is not considered here. Left atrioventricular valve stenosis is also sometimes seen following repair of atrioventricular septal defects. Whatever the cause, obstruction to mitral inflow leads to an elevated left atrial pressure which is transmitted to the pulmonary veins leading to pulmonary hypertension.

History

As with all valvar lesions, if the degree of mitral stenosis is mild there will be no symptoms and the only signs will be on auscultation. As noted, congenital mitral stenosis may coexist with left heart obstruction at aortic valvar level and with coarctation and the prognosis depends upon the whole complex. As the degree of stenosis and/or regurgitation progresses, effort dyspnoea will develop. There will also be orthopnoea and paroxysmal cough, as well as a susceptibility to chest infections. Syncope can be a symptom of mitral stenosis and adults may have haemoptysis. Pulmonary hypertension may cause dilatation of the pulmonary trunk and pressure on the recurrent laryngeal nerve leading to a hoarse voice. The rate of progression of the disease will vary but in severe cases symptoms of congestive cardiac failure will develop.

Examination

The so-called 'mitral facies' is a feature of chronic severe mitral stenosis. In chronic mitral stenosis, atrial fibrillation or flutter may occur. An atrial communication may coexist with mitral stenosis, and lead to an elevated JVP. Without an atrial communication, the JVP is elevated due to pulmonary hypertension. This pulmonary hypertension, also leads to a prominent right ventricular impulse and a loud second sound. There is a diastolic murmur best heard at the apex and in severe cases of mitral stenosis there may be an apical *diastolic* thrill that is easy to mistime as systolic without careful comparison with a central pulse.

Heart sounds	Loud S_1 Loud S_2 (if pulmonary hypertension)
Added sounds	Opening snap, S_4
Murmurs	Mitral stenosis: apical mid-diastolic, rumbling with presystolic accentuation (if sinus rhythm) Mitral regurgitation: apical long or pansystolic murmur Murmur of pulmonary regurgitation and/or tricuspid regurgitation if severe pulmonary hypertension supervenes

ECG

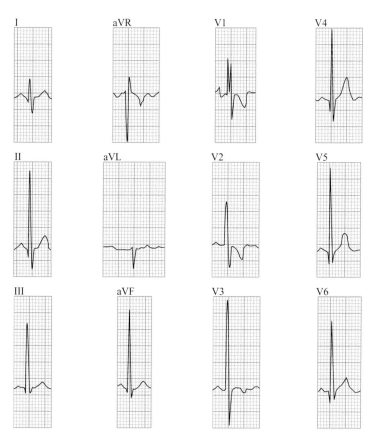

Fig. 6.4 *This patient has moderate mitral stenosis. In this ECG the P wave duration is increased, and in lead V1 there is a large late negative deflection. These findings are typical of left atrial hypertrophy. Incidentally, there is incomplete right bundle branch block (normal QRS duration, with RSR¹ pattern in lead V1)*

The ECG is usually abnormal in significant mitral stenosis. There is generally evidence of left atrial hypertrophy, and if pulmonary hypertension supervenes there will be voltage criteria for right ventricular hypertrophy. In adults there may be atrial fibrillation or flutter.

CXR

This may be normal in very mild disease. Significant disease will cause prominence of the left atrium with splaying of the carina. Pulmonary venous hypertension will be reflected by prominent upper lobe veins. The enlarged left atrium causes prominence of the appendage and straightening of the left heart border. There may be calcification in the region of the mitral valve, notably in rheumatic mitral stenosis. In severe disease, as pulmonary arterial hypertension develops, there will be prominence of the central pulmonary arteries with, in advanced cases, peripheral arterial pruning.

Echocardiogram

The anatomy of the mitral valve is assessed. The gradient across the mitral valve, effective valve orifice and pulmonary pressure are all assessed. The presence or absence of an atrial communication is noted.

Notes

The opening snap and loud first heart sound depend upon a mobile valve leaflet, and although heard in rheumatic mitral stenosis, may be absent in congenital forms of mitral stenosis, depending on the morphology of the valve. The murmurs of mitral valve disease are loudest at the apex and are accentuated by laying the patient on the left side and listening with the bell of the stethoscope.

In a case of mixed mitral disease it is important to be able to make an assessment of the haemodynamic importance of each: if the dominant lesion is stenosis, the heart will not be enlarged on palpation, there may be a diastolic thrill, the P_2 may be palpable, and the murmur will be loudest in diastole. Don't forget the late diastolic (pre-systolic) accentuation caused by the active phase of left ventricular filling secondary to atrial systole. This is lost if the patient is not in sinus rhythm.

If the dominant lesion is regurgitation, the apex will be displaced and thrusting and the dominant murmur will be systolic. Remember that if regurgitation is important the diastolic murmur may be accentuated because of the resulting increased diastolic flow across the mitral valve: a mitral diastolic murmur can even develop when there is no stenosis (see mitral regurgitation above).

Pulmonary hypertension may lead to a pansystolic murmur of tricuspid regurgitation, and the dilated right ventricle and small left ventricle may make this move more towards the apex than is usual. There will however be an increase in volume on inspiration that should differentiate this from mitral regurgitation.

Learning points

- It is possible to assess which lesion is dominant in mixed mitral valve disease
- A *diastolic* thrill in mitral stenosis is easy to mistime as *systolic*

Summary		
● Where is the murmur loudest?	→	Apex
● When does the murmur occur?	→	Diastole (stenosis) and systole (regurgitation)
● What else could it be?	→	Nothing
● What makes it mitral stenosis and mitral regurgitation?	→	Timing and position of the murmur

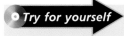 **6.3 Mitral stenosis and regurgitation**

- Now listen to the mitral stenosis and regurgitation recording on the CD. Use the suggestions to ensure that you have identified the systolic and diastolic murmurs. This is a recording made at the apex in a patient with mitral stenosis and regurgitation. The systolic murmur is due to mild mitral regurgitation and the diastolic murmur is mild mitral stenosis. Try to time the sounds with the SDC. The mitral regurgitation obviously coincides with the SDC hitting systole, and the mitral stenosis with the cursor hitting diastole. When you feel that you have identified the systolic and diastolic murmurs, minimize diastole. This causes S_1 to be very soft and S_2 prominent. Listen to the systolic murmur for a few cycles and note that there is nothing after S_2 (during diastole). When you feel that you are confident maximize diastole. You have now enhanced the diastolic mitral stenosis murmur and can hopefully hear it more easily than in the native recording. It is described as low pitched and rumbling. Repeat the last two steps, minimizing and maximizing diastole until you can confidently hear the mitral stenosis murmur. You may also be able to appreciate the presystolic accentuation caused by atrial systole just before S_1.

- If you are still unsure that you have identified the diastolic murmur minimize systole. This removes the systolic murmur so only the diastolic murmur is left and this is at maximum intensity. Finally listen to the native recording and be clear of the two separate murmurs.

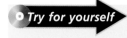

- Now listen to the recording of the opening snap in mitral stenosis. Use the suggestions to ensure that you have identified the correct sound. This is a recording of pure mild mitral stenosis and from the apex. The first heart sound S_1 is loud but the diastolic murmur of mitral stenosis in this case is soft. The opening snap is a prominent feature. Time the sounds with the SDC. The opening snap follows very soon after S_2 and can indeed be confused with splitting of S_2. When you have listened to the native murmur, minimize diastole, which will eliminate both the opening snap and the soft diastolic murmur.

- S_1 remains prominent and S_2 is soft. Listen to the sound for a few cycles and note that there is nothing after S_2 (during diastole). Watch the SDC while listening. Get the timing of each part of the cardiac cycle.

- Next maximize diastole which accentuates the opening snap after S_2 and the diastolic murmur which immediately follows it. Repeat these two steps, minimizing and maximizing diastole until you are confident that you can hear the opening snap and the murmur. When you are confident, listen again to the native murmur, you should now be able to appreciate clearly the opening snap, although the diastolic murmur is soft.

Quiz

The following statements are true or false. Cover the answers to test your understanding.

1. Worldwide, rheumatic fever is the commonest cause of mitral stenosis.
2. There may be an apical systolic thrill in mitral stenosis.
3. There is always presystolic accentuation of mitral stenosis murmur.
4. Mitral stenosis and regurgitation may coexist.
5. Bacterial endocarditis may further damage a stenotic mitral valve.
6. Calcification of the mitral valve may be seen on CXR in MS.
7. An opening snap is common in congenital mitral stenosis.
8. A pulmonary regurgitation murmur may coexist with severe MS.
9. The ECG is usually normal in moderate mitral stenosis.
10. Mitral stenosis may coexist with an atrial communication.

Answers to quiz

1. True, although rheumatic fever is now uncommon in developed countries, worldwide it is still the commonest cause of MS.
2. False. The apical thrill is diastolic, although it can be easy to mistime it.
3. False. This depends upon the patient being in sinus rhythm, and atrial fibrillation is a common complication of mitral stenosis.
4. True. The balance between MR and MS may alter over time.
5. True. Endocarditis will generally lead to worsening regurgitation.
6. True. Rheumatic mitral stenosis may lead to calcification and fibrosis of the valve as the condition progresses.
7. False. An opening snap is more common in rheumatic disease, and less common when the valve is congenitally abnormal.
8. True. Mitral stenosis leads to pulmonary hypertension and so may produce audible pulmonary regurgitation.
9. False. The ECG will usually show signs of left atrial hypertrophy, and may show right ventricular hypertrophy if there is PHT.
10. True. The presence of an atrial communication will lessen the left atrial pressure, and so the pulmonary hypertension, but will lead to a decreased systemic cardiac output.

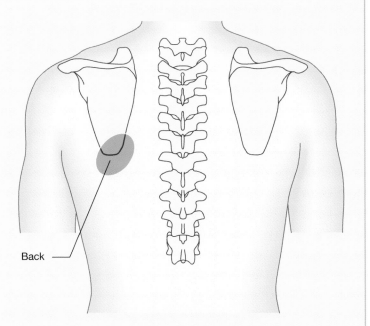

Back

A few murmurs are not just transmitted to the back of the chest but are actually louder there

The murmurs best heard at the back are:

- Coarctation
- Branch pulmonary artery stenosis

Coarctation

Anatomy

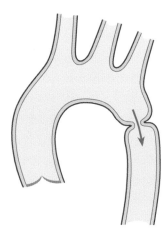

Fig. 7.1 *Coarctation*

Coarctation of the aorta may be an isolated abnormality or may be associated with abnormalities of the aortic valve, mitral valve and the aortic arch. A patent ductus arteriosus is not unusual, particularly in the infant form, and a VSD may also coexist. The coarctation may be due to a 'shelf', or a fibrous ring may encircle the aorta. This occurs at the level of insertion of the ductus arteriosus or the ductal ligament if the duct is shut. There may be long tubular narrowing of the aortic arch and this may be in addition to a coarctation 'shelf' or may be an isolated abnormality. The left subclavian artery may be narrowed by the coarctation. Abdominal aortic coarctation is much rarer than the thoracic form and is usually an acquired condition in association with a systemic vascular disorder such as Takayasu arteritis.

History

There are more males than females affected by coarctation. Coarctation may present in the neonatal period or early infancy with collapse and in this situation associated left heart abnormalities are common and a specific murmur from the coarctation site is usually absent, either because of the presence of a patent ductus arteriosus, or because there is very little flow through the site of the coarctation. Patients presenting after the first year of life will often be asymptomatic, symptoms if present will usually be as a result of associated hypertension, and include heart failure, dissection of the aorta and cerebral haemorrhage. Some patients complain of leg fatigue, or cold feet, but these symptoms are common in the normal population. There is an increased risk of bacterial endocarditis.

Examination

Coarctation of the aorta is more common in Turner's syndrome, and features of this should be sought. Palpation of the femoral pulses will show low volume or completely absent pulses. The left brachial pulse may be normal or low volume depending on the relationship of the coarctation to the left subclavian artery and an associated abnormal origin of the right subclavian artery may affect the right arm pulses. There may be visible pulsation in the neck and a suprasternal thrill. The blood pressure will often be elevated in the right arm. The apex may be forceful in the older patient with coarctation, but in the neonate a right ventricular impulse is felt because of pulmonary hypertension.

Heart sounds	*Normal*
Added sounds	*Nil, unless associated with valvar heart disease*
Murmurs	*Ejection systolic murmur over posterior left side of chest; continuous murmur over posterior chest wall (collaterals)*

ECG

This will often be normal but may show left ventricular hypertrophy because of upper body hypertension. In neonates there may be right ventricular hypertrophy because of pulmonary hypertension.

CXR

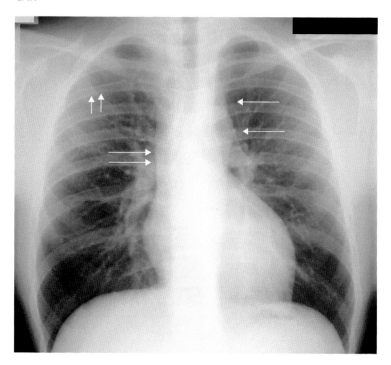

Fig. 7.2 *Coarctation of the aorta. There are a number of features confirming coarctation of the aorta. There is the 'reverse 3' sign: the top arrow represents the aorta just above the coarctation and the bottom one indicates the dilated aorta just below it (so-called post-stenotic dilatation). The ascending aorta is also prominent (double arrows), and the rounded contour of the left heart border suggests left ventricular hypertrophy (these patients are usually hypertensive). There is rib notching due to dilatation of the intercostals arteries*

The chest X-ray may be normal in mild disease. There may be cardiomegaly, either due to left ventricular hypertrophy, or left ventricular dilatation from chronic pressure overload. The aortic arch shadow may be inconspicuous. There may be a '3 sign'; at the left upper border there is prominence of the arch just proximal to the narrow segment and post-stenotic dilatation just beyond. In adults and older children with good collateral arterial supply there may be rib notching.

Echocardiogram

Echocardiogram will define the anatomy and severity of the coarctation in younger patients, however in older subjects other imaging, such as angiography or cardiac MRI, may be superior.

Notes

There will often be an aortic ejection click at the apex, possibly with an aortic systolic murmur due to the frequent association of a bicuspid aortic valve. Hypertension in coarctation is not simply related to the obstruction because it may persist despite good surgical correction. The aorta proximal to the coarctation is stiffer than the normal aorta and less distensible, so the normal systolic rise in blood pressure on exercise is enhanced. The carotid sinus baroreceptors are reset at a higher level in coarctation. There is also a renal component, and hypertension is induced if there is aortic narrowing proximal to the renal arteries.

Cerebral haemorrhage in coarctation is not just the result of hypertension, but occurs because of associated intracranial aneurysms.

In tight coarctation the posterior murmur through the coarctation may be continuous.

Summary	
● Where is the murmur loudest?	→ At the back
● When does the murmur occur?	→ Systole
● What else could it be?	→ Branch pulmonary artery stenosis
● What makes it coarctation?	→ Presence of poor femoral pulses

● Try for yourself 7.1 Coarctation

● Now listen to the coarctation recording on the CD. Initially listen to the native sound and try to appreciate the systolic murmur. If you are having trouble, initially minimize systole. This has abolished the murmur. After listening for a few cardiac cycles, maximize systole. This makes the murmur more prominent. Repeat these two steps until you are confident that you can hear the murmur. Finally reset and listen to the native murmur.

Quiz

The following statements about coarctation of the aorta are true or false. Answer them and then check the answers below.

1. Coarctation of the aorta is more common in males.
2. Patients with coarctation are usually identified from typical symptoms.
3. Coarctation may be diagnosed on chest X-ray.
4. The coarctation murmur is best heard at the back.
5. Coarctation is rarely associated with bacterial endocarditis.
6. Hypertension in coarctation is abolished if the obstruction is successfully relieved.
7. Coarctation may present with an intracranial haemorrhage.
8. Coarctation may present with severe chest pain.
9. Coarctation in a neonate will usually be accompanied by left ventricular hypertrophy on the ECG.
10. Coarctation should be considered in all cases of systemic hypertension.

Answers to quiz

1. True. Estimates of the ratio vary from 1.3 to 1 to 3 to 1.
2. False. Like many forms of structural heart disease, the patient is often asymptomatic, even in the presence of significant disease.
3. True. The presence of a 3 sign is diagnostic of coarctation.
4. True. It is best heard just to the left of the spine at the back.
5. False. The endocarditis may be at the site of the coarctation, or may occur on a coexisting bicuspid aortic valve.
6. False. Because of the abnormalities in the aortic wall and vascular bed in patients with coarctation, abnormal hypertension, particularly systolic hypertension often persists despite successful relief of the obstruction.
7. True. This is due to associated intracranial aneurysms, as well as systemic hypertension.
8. True. The aorta may dissect at its arch, at the coarctation site, or because of a mycotic aneurysm.
9. False. In neonates, right ventricular hypertrophy is more common because of pulmonary hypertension.
10. True. Although it is more likely to be a cause in a relatively young person, since it can be excluded simply by feeling the femoral pulse, it should be considered in all cases.

Branch pulmonary artery stenosis

Anatomy

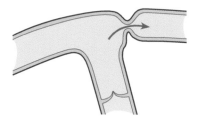

Fig. 7.3 *Branch pulmonary artery stenosis*

In the newborn infant, particularly premature babies and those who are small at birth, it is very common to hear a murmur arising from the origin of either pulmonary artery. This occurs because during fetal life the majority of the blood exiting the right ventricle crosses the patent ductus arteriosus to the descending aorta. After birth, with the closure of the arterial duct, the whole right ventricular output goes to the lungs and the branch pulmonary arteries grow to accommodate this over the first few months of life.

True narrowings at the origins of either pulmonary artery, or further out in the pulmonary arterial tree, are relatively frequent in association with tetralogy of Fallot. Pulmonary arterial abnormalities may also occur in association with Williams syndrome, Alagille syndrome and fetal rubella.

History

Patients will often be asymptomatic, although breathlessness on exertion may be a feature with important narrowing.

Examination

Facial appearance of the patient may suggest a syndrome, such as Williams, and a thorough general examination to elicit features is necessary. If the stenoses are associated with tetralogy of Fallot, or are severe and in the presence of an atrial septal defect, there may be central cyanosis. Bilateral, severe stenoses may lead to signs of right ventricular hypertrophy, with a right ventricular heave, and eventually right ventricular failure, with a raised jugular venous pressure, hepatomegaly and peripheral oedema.

Heart sounds	*Normal*
Added sounds	*Nil*
Murmurs	*Ejection systolic murmur over the affected lung(s)*

ECG
There may be signs of right ventricular hypertrophy, although these may be absent, even in the presence of a significantly raised right ventricular pressure.

CXR
If the stenosis is unilateral, there may be a difference in the pulmonary vascular markings visible on comparing the two lungs. In multiple peripheral stenoses, the overall pulmonary vascularity may be decreased. The cardiac contour is often normal until the onset of right ventricular failure.

Echocardiogram
Echocardiogram will show turbulence in the branch pulmonary artery, and allow an estimate of right ventricular pressure to be obtained. Other cardiac abnormalities, such as atrial or ventricular septal defects will be shown. For multiple, peripheral pulmonary artery narrowings pulmonary angiography is superior.

Notes

Branch pulmonary artery murmurs are often audible over the whole precordium, but are louder posteriorly over the lung fields. Rarely, there may be a diastolic component due to diastolic forward flow in severe cases. The murmurs are crescendo decrescendo and may begin relatively late in the cardiac cycle. Occasionally continuous murmurs may be heard over the lung fields in severe branch pulmonary artery stenosis, and these arise from bronchial collateral arteries. Branch pulmonary artery stenosis may be acquired, for example, due to pressure on the left pulmonary artery from a device to close a patent ductus arteriosus.

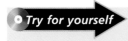 **Try for yourself** ▸ **7.2 Branch pulmonary
artery stenosis**

- Now listen to the recording of branch pulmonary artery stenosis on the CD.
  This was recorded at the back on the left. There is a systolic murmur audible.
  Once you have listened to the murmur, minimize systole and listen again. The
  murmur has been abolished. Next, maximize systole. The murmur is now
  louder and easier to appreciate. Repeat these two steps minimizing and
  maximizing systole until you are confident that you have identified the
  murmur. Finally, listen to the native murmur and be sure that you can identify
  the branch pulmonary artery murmur.

Quiz

The following statements about branch pulmonary stenosis are true or false. Try to answer them all and then check with the answers below.

1. Branch pulmonary artery murmurs are common in preterm babies.
2. Branch pulmonary artery murmurs are heard more easily over the precordium.
3. There may be continuous murmurs on branch pulmonary artery stenosis.
4. Branch pulmonary artery stenosis may occur with tetralogy of Fallot.
5. The ECG may be normal with branch pulmonary artery stenosis.
6. Patients with branch pulmonary artery stenosis are not cyanosed.
7. The chest X-ray is not helpful in the assessment of branch pulmonary artery stenosis.
8. Branch pulmonary artery stenosis may be treated by cardiac catheter intervention.
9. Branch pulmonary artery stenosis may occur in congenital rubella infection.
10. Branch pulmonary artery stenosis may be asymptomatic.

Answers to quiz

1. True. The majority disappear within 6 months as the pulmonary arteries grow.
2. False. They are most easily heard over the back and in the axillae.
3. True. Most probably arising from collateral arteries.
4. True. Branch pulmonary artery abnormalities are common in tetralogy of Fallot.
5. True. This may be the case with quite severe disease.
6. False. An atrial communication is a reasonably common association and may lead to cyanosis.
7. False. The chest X-ray can be very helpful, particularly in unilateral stenosis.
8. True. The narrowings may be ballooned or stented.
9. True. Also in Williams and Allagille syndromes.
10. True, although effort intolerance may occur in moderate to severe disease.

Glossary

Apex: The apex of the heart is the most lateral and caudal point on the chest where the cardiac pulsation may be felt.

Arrhythmia: Abnormally fast or slow heart rate.

Ascites: Free fluid in the abdominal cavity. May occur in severe cardiac failure.

Bell chestpiece: Part of stethoscope designed to detect low frequency sounds.

Cyanosis: Blueness. This may be peripheral, affecting the extremities, which is normal in the cold and is common in children, or central, affecting the lips and tongue as well as the extremities, and indicates a low arterial oxygen tension.

Dependent oedema: Swelling which due to gravity affects the lowest part of the body. In mobile individuals this will be the ankles, but in bedridden patients this may be the sacrum.

Dextrocardia: Situation when the apex of the heart is in the right chest.

Diabetes: Abnormality of glucose metabolism that is associated with an increased risk of cardiovascular disease.

Diaphragm chestpiece: Part of stethoscope designed to detect high frequency sounds.

Down's syndrome: Also known as trisomy 21. Condition in which there is an extra chromosome 21. It is associated with structural cardiac abnormalities, as well as learning difficulties, gut and joint problems.

Dysmorphic: Unusual features, such as single palmar creases, or facial features.

Ejection: Sound caused by the heart ejecting blood in systole. May either be a click from a valve opening, or a murmur from blood passing through the valve.

Finger clubbing: A loss of the normal angle between the nail bed and the skin progressing to a bulbous swelling of the terminal phalanges. This may also affect the toes. It may be congenital, or associated with cardiac, pulmonary, liver or gut disease.

First heart sound: The sound caused by the closure of the mitral and tricuspid valves.

Hypertension: High blood pressure. Definition depends upon age and the context of the measurement.

Intercostal: Between the ribs.

Lipid status: Level of cholesterol and triglycerides in the blood. Abnormally high levels or imbalances may predispose to cardiovascular disease.

Marfan syndrome: Condition due to abnormality of collagen which is characterized by tall stature, hypermobility of the joint, and may involve lens dislocation and cardiac involvement with mitral valve prolapse and aortic root dilatation or rupture.

Mitral valve: The valve between the left atrium and the left ventricle in a structurally normal heart.

Myxomatous: Jelly-like thickening of a valve.

Obesity: Excess fatty tissue.

Orthopnoea: Breathlessness on lying flat. This may be due to cardiac or pulmonary disease.

Palpitations: An awareness of the heartbeat in the chest.

Paroxysmal nocturnal dyspnoea: Breathlessness which wakens a patient from sleep and is relieved by sitting up. It may be associated with a cough and frothy or lightly blood stained sputum.

Pericardial effusion: Collection of fluid between the two layers of pericardium which may compromise the function of the heart.

Pericardium: The two-layered sac which surrounds the heart.

Phonocardiogram: A recording of heart sounds.

Pleural effusions: Excess fluid present between the two layers of the pleura.

Regurgitation: Leaking of a valve.

Second heart sound: The sound caused by the closure of the aortic and pulmonary valves.

Sphygmomanometer: Device for measuring blood pressure.

Stenosis: Narrowing of a valve.

Stethoscope: Acoustic instrument which allows transmission and amplification of the heart sounds from the chest wall to the listener.

Syncope: Symptom. Sudden loss of consciousness.

Systole: Phase of the cardiac cycle. Usually refers to ventricular systole, but the atrial systole is during the last third of ventricular diastole. When referring to blood pressure, this means the higher reading.

Systemic: Pertaining to the body.

Tachycardia: Fast heart rate. Depends on age (children have faster heart rates than adults). May be sinus, i.e. normal, or due to an arrhythmia, i.e. abnormal.

Tricuspid valve: The valve between the right atrium and the right ventricle in a structurally normal heart.

Valsalva manoeuvre: Raising intrathoracic and intra-abdominal pressure by exhaling against a closed glottis. Occurs during childbirth, and when straining to defecate.

Vasovagal: Applied to syncope or bradycardia caused by overactivity of the vaso-vagal nerve.

Xanthomata: Yellow or orange deposits of lipid in the skin. Around the eyes these are known as xanthelasma, and may be normal in the elderly.

Index

Page numbers in **bold** represent main discussions. Those in *italics* refer to CD tutorials.

ELSEVIER CD-ROM LICENCE AGREEMENT

PLEASE READ THE FOLLOWING AGREEMENT CAREFULLY BEFORE USING THIS PRODUCT. THIS PRODUCT IS LICENSED UNDER THE TERMS CONTAINED IN THIS LICENCE AGREEMENT ('Agreement'). BY USING THIS PRODUCT, YOU, AN INDIVIDUAL OR ENTITY INCLUDING EMPLOYEES, AGENTS AND REPRESENTATIVES ('You' or 'Your'), ACKNOWLEDGE THAT YOU HAVE READ THIS AGREEMENT, THAT YOU UNDERSTAND IT, AND THAT YOU AGREE TO BE BOUND BY THE TERMS AND CONDITIONS OF THIS AGREEMENT. ELSEVIER LIMITED ('Elsevier') EXPRESSLY DOES NOT AGREE TO LICENSE THIS PRODUCT TO YOU UNLESS YOU ASSENT TO THIS AGREEMENT. IF YOU DO NOT AGREE WITH ANY OF THE FOLLOWING TERMS, YOU MAY, WITHIN THIRTY (30) DAYS AFTER YOUR RECEIPT OF THIS PRODUCT RETURN THE UNUSED PRODUCT AND ALL ACCOMPANYING DOCUMENTATION TO ELSEVIER FOR A FULL REFUND.

DEFINITIONS As used in this Agreement, these terms shall have the following meanings:

'Proprietary Material' means the valuable and proprietary information content of this Product including without limitation all indexes and graphic materials and software used to access, index, search and retrieve the information content from this Product developed or licensed by Elsevier and/or its affiliates, suppliers and licensors.

'Product' means the copy of the Proprietary Material and any other material delivered on CD-ROM and any other human readable or machine-readable materials enclosed with this Agreement, including without limitation documentation relating to the same.

OWNERSHIP This Product has been supplied by and is proprietary to Elsevier and/or its affiliates, suppliers and licensors. The copyright in the Product belongs to Elsevier and/or its affiliates, suppliers and licensors and is protected by the copyright, trademark, trade secret and other intellectual property laws of the United Kingdom and international treaty provisions, including without limitation the Universal Copyright Convention and the Berne Copyright Convention. You have no ownership rights in this Product. Except as expressly set forth herein, no part of this Product, including without limitation the Proprietary Material, may be modified, copied or distributed in hardcopy or machine-readable form without prior written consent from Elsevier. All rights not expressly granted to You herein are expressly reserved. Any other use of this Product by any person or entity is strictly prohibited and a violation of this Agreement.

SCOPE OF RIGHTS LICENSED (PERMITTED USES) Elsevier is granting to You a limited, non-exclusive, non-transferable licence to use this Product in accordance with the terms of this Agreement. You may use or provide access to this Product on a single computer or terminal physically located at Your premises and in a secure network or move this Product to and use it on another single computer or terminal at the same location for personal use only, but under no circumstances may You use or provide access to any part or parts of this Product on more than one computer or terminal simultaneously.

You shall not (a) copy, download, or otherwise reproduce the Product or any part(s) thereof in any medium, including, without limitation, online transmissions, local area networks, wide area networks, intranets, extranets and the Internet, or in any way, in whole or in part, except for printing out or downloading nonsubstantial portions of the text and images in the Product for Your own personal use; (b) alter, modify, or adapt the Product or any part(s) thereof, including but not limited to decompiling, disassembling, reverse engineering, or creating derivative works, without the prior written approval of Elsevier; (c) sell, license or otherwise distribute to third parties the Product or any part(s) thereof; or (d) alter, remove, obscure or obstruct the display of any copyright, trademark or other proprietary notice on or in the Product or on any printout or download of portions of the Proprietary Materials.

RESTRICTIONS ON TRANSFER This Licence is personal to You, and neither Your rights hereunder nor the tangible embodiments of this Product, including without limitation the Proprietary Material, may be sold, assigned, transferred or sublicensed to any other person, including without limitation by operation of law, without the prior written consent of Elsevier. Any purported sale, assignment, transfer or sublicense without the prior written consent of Elsevier will be void and will automatically terminate the Licence granted hereunder.

TERM This Agreement will remain in effect until terminated pursuant to the terms of this Agreement. You may terminate this Agreement at any time by removing from Your system and destroying the Product and any copies of the Proprietary Material. Unauthorized copying of the Product, including without limitation, the Proprietary Material and documentation, or otherwise failing to comply with the terms and conditions of this Agreement shall result in automatic termination of this licence and will make available to Elsevier legal remedies. Upon termination of this Agreement, the licence granted herein will terminate and You must immediately destroy the Product and all copies of the Product and of the Proprietary Material, together with any and all accompanying documentation. All provisions relating to proprietary rights shall survive termination of this Agreement.

LIMITED WARRANTY AND LIMITATION OF LIABILITY Elsevier warrants that the software embodied in this Product will perform in substantial compliance with the documentation supplied in this Product, unless the performance problems are the result of hardware failure or improper use. If You report a significant defect in performance in writing to Elsevier within ninety (90) calendar days of your having purchased the Product, and Elsevier is not able to correct same within sixty (60) days after its receipt of Your notification, You may return this Product, including all copies and documentation, to Elsevier and Elsevier will refund Your money. In order to apply for a refund on your purchased Product, please contact the return address on the invoice to obtain the refund request form ('Refund Request Form'), and either fax or mail your signed request and your proof of purchase to the address indicated on the Refund Request Form. Incomplete forms will not be processed. Defined terms in the Refund Request Form shall have the same meaning as in this Agreement.